"Caroline Frizell gives us a thought-provoking perspective of eco-feminist dance movement psychotherapy. This is a beautifully written book that offers an extraordinary resource to anyone wanting to understand the intrinsic therapeutic power of dance, movement and eco-psychotherapy practices, explored through the lens of social, political, and environmental justice."
– **Professor Claudia Bernard**, *Goldsmiths, University of London*

"This book entices you through peristaltic rhythms with perfect pacing and deliciously textured writing rooting and spreading through diverse ecologies. The author's lived experience is made tangible as she weaves the connective tissues of human and more-than-human bodies placing the whole earth as both core and container."
– **Penelope A Best/O.Pen Be**, *Eco-active Live Artist, DMP practitioner, International Facilitator of Relational Creative Practice (RCPM)*

"This book is genuinely accessible in engaging with academic philosophies and practices of new materialism, posthumanism, critical disability studies and intersectionality as lenses for re-envisioning dance movement psychotherapy. I see readers on a park bench absorbed in this book: students, researchers, parents, teachers, those interested in ecology, disability, equality and how we create a fairer world."
– **Roz Carroll**, *Co-editor of What is normal? Psychotherapists explore the question'*

"This beautifully written text dances between poetic prose and client-therapist relationship framed by critical theory. The journey from sea to therapy room invites us to notice and find gold in the ordinary. This book is about inclusion, difference and staying with the trouble; a must-read for anyone in the healing professions."
– **Mary-Jayne Rust**, *Ecopsychotherapist, and author of Towards and Ecopsychotherapy.*

"Frizell's writing will catapult you from profound philosophical ideas to moments of stillness; bringing into focus the everyday-taken-for-granted treasures of our relational rhizomatic aliveness-in-the-world. Whether you have come to it as therapist, dance practitioner, researcher, philosopher, educator, health professional, activist or an interested bystander, this book will change you in multiple ways."
– **Marina Rova**, *PhD: mover, cultural nomad, earth traveller and co-editor of 'Creative Bodies in Therapy, Performance and Community. Research and Practice that Brings Us Home' (Routledge 2023).*

"What a relief to read academic research so present to the encounter between . . . not just persons, not just chairs but the world outside listening-in. It is like van Gogh's shoes – very ordinary with an inner radiance of aliveness. The pearl is in the rabid imagining."

– **Chris Robertson**, *co-founder of Re-Vision psychotherapy training and climate psychology author.*

"In being invited into the folds of Frizell's creative explorations, I understand more about the landscapes I roam in ways that, paradoxically, are suddenly a little nonsensical. Well-trodden patterns are a bit befuddled and the parts of me that want to 'stay with the trouble' are thrilled."

– **Emma Palmer**, *Relational Body Psychotherapist, ecopsychologist, supervisor, facilitator and writer. Bristol, UK*

"A beautiful, intricately woven and profoundly embodied gift of love and presence – to the earth and all her beings. Compassionate and extraordinarily sensitive, finely detailed yet huge in vision, breadth and inclusion."

– **Hilary Prentice**, *retired psychotherapist and sometime ecopsychology pioneer.*

"This book holds the reader *alive* in the phenomenological here and now relationships to all that surrounds us. Individual human and more than human subjects have value and impact in the intra-connectedness of Frizell's narrative, with inclusivity as an essential mycorrhizal connection for the human and more than human."

– **Geoffery Unkovich**, *Dance Movement Psychotherapist, Supervisor, and Senior Lecturer for UK universities and European training programmes.*

"Frizell celebrates the extraordinary in the ordinary in this skilfully crafted assemblage. It is an ode to the dance of life; provocative and reassuring all at once. Dance movement psychotherapy is considered through intimate accounts where the personal is professional and the professional is political. Be unsettled. Let this book awaken your attention."

– **Céline Butée**, *UKCP HIPC & ADMP-UK Registered Dance Movement Psychotherapist, Supervisor & Training Supervisor, Dancer.*

Posthuman Possibilities of Dance Movement Psychotherapy

This timely book explores an ecofeminist approach to dance movement psychotherapy, with an emphasis on the posthuman possibilities of differently enabled bodies and fostering social, political and environmental justice.

Using the lenses of posthumanism and new materialism, this book examines the points of convergence among dance movement psychotherapy, ecopsychotherapy and critical disability studies. It maps out the experience of building care, empathy and kinship and explores ecologically informed, embodied practices and research, while offering new perspectives on these practices. Structured using thematic 'interruptions' between chapters to anchor the reading experience and provide coherence, chapters include case study extracts as examples from the practices, spanning group work and individual therapy with autistic and learning-disabled children and young people, as well as with neurotypical adult clients in private practice.

Bringing together practice and research in dance movement psychotherapy along with cutting-edge theoretical perspectives of new materialism and posthumanism, the book will be of great interest to researchers and students of dance therapy, arts therapies, ecopsychotherapy and disability studies. It will also be useful to practitioners and therapists in psychotherapy and well-being services.

Caroline Frizell is Senior Lecturer in Dance Movement Psychotherapy at Goldsmiths, University of London, UK, and an ecologically informed dance movement psychotherapist, supervisor and author.

Routledge Research in Creative Arts and Expressive Therapies

This series provides a forum to discuss the latest research, debates and practice in creative arts and expressive therapies, including arts therapy, dance therapy, dramatherapy and music therapy.

Intercultural Music Therapy Consultation Research
Shared Humanity in Collaborative Theory and Practice
Lisa Margetts

Reflections on Authentic Movement
Theory, Practice and Arts-Led Research
Eila Goldhahn

Space, Place and Dramatherapy
International Perspectives
Edited by Eliza Sweeney

Posthuman Possibilities of Dance Movement Psychotherapy
Moving through Ecofeminist and New Materialist Entanglements of Differently Enabled Bodies in Research
Caroline Frizell

Posthuman Possibilities of Dance Movement Psychotherapy

Moving through Ecofeminist and New Materialist Entanglements of Differently Enabled Bodies in Research

Caroline Frizell

R Routledge
Taylor & Francis Group

LONDON AND NEW YORK

First published 2024
by Routledge
4 Park Square, Milton Park, Abingdon, Oxon OX14 4RN

and by Routledge
605 Third Avenue, New York, NY 10158

Routledge is an imprint of the Taylor & Francis Group, an informa business

© 2024 Caroline Frizell

British Library Cataloguing-in-Publication Data
A catalogue record for this book is available from the British Library

Library of Congress Cataloging-in-Publication Data
Names: Frizell, Caroline, author.
Title: Posthuman possibilities of dance movement psychotherapy : moving through eco-feminist and new materialist entanglements of differently enabled bodies in research / Caroline Frizell. Abingdon, Oxon ; New York, NY : Routledge, 2024.
Series: Routledge research in creative arts and expressive therapies | Includes bibliographical references and index.
Identifiers: LCCN 2023021326 (print) | LCCN 2023021327 (ebook) | ISBN 9781032345352 (hbk) | ISBN 9781032345376 (pbk) | ISBN 9781003322658 (ebk)
Subjects: LCSH: Dance therapy. | Ecofeminism. | Environmental psychology.
Classification: LCC RC489.D3 F753 2024 (print) | LCC RC489.D3 (ebook) | DDC 616.89/1655—dc23/eng/20230724
LC record available at https://lccn.loc.gov/2023021326
LC ebook record available at https://lccn.loc.gov/2023021327

ISBN: 978-1-032-34535-2 (hbk)
ISBN: 978-1-032-34537-6 (pbk)
ISBN: 978-1-003-32265-8 (ebk)

DOI: 10.4324/9781003322658

Contents

Acknowledgements

This book materialised with the support and love of some remarkable presences in this world.

Alan, Anna, Amelia and Esther, thank you for the decades of fun, love, laughter and inspiration that made this book possible. I am also indebted to my late mother, Georgina, who gifted me a love of dance, and my father, Leslie, who filled my life with literary appreciation and sadly died in the year of his centenary, just before I finished this book. Thérèse Moody, my dancing comrade, who was taken from this earth too soon; your spirit lives on in this endeavour. Dr Farhad Dalal, thanks for the loyalty and encouragement, and thanks to all other colleagues who make for an inspirational community. My gratitude also goes to the wisteria who blooms outside the window in the summer, the laurel who stays green all year and the blue tit who nests in the streetlight in spring. To the parliament of rooks and their noisy social gatherings. To bees, wasps and flies who pass by the window and the sun that creeps around to my office window in the afternoons. To the blue sky and the scudding clouds. Thanks also to Dartmoor, for allowing me to move with you and for the inspiration offered by the landscape. To Strete, Mothecombe and Start Point; to St Ives and Zennor, the shifting tides and the wisdom of the more-than-human.

Figures

List of terms

A transversal perspective on terminologies and concepts that cuts across disciplines.

Ableism is a discrimination against disabled people within an ability/disability binary that marginalises and subordinates disability.

Activism is any action that endeavours to influence policy, research and practice in social, political and environmental justice.

Advanced capitalism is an economic system driven by competition and profit that has become embedded in social, cultural, economic and political structures.

Affect is an intra-active, relational intensity between the component parts of an assemblage created by constituent entities affecting and being affected from multiple vertices. This expands the psychoanalytic notion of affect as (human) emotional and mental phenomena linked to pleasure and gratification. Posthumanism and new materialism move beyond the idea that human affectivity is paramount towards a notion of humans as part of a wider affective economy within an intra-active living world.

Affect economy refers to dynamic processes by which component parts of an assemblage affect each other from within, creating an always-in-process production of knowledge (Fox & Alldred, 2015), with an orientation towards 'processes and flows rather than structures and stable forms' (407).

Agential realism troubles the idea that agency is a human prerogative in which humans have agency over other inert, albeit considered animate or inanimate, life.

Anthropocene is an era in which human activity has had a significant and often a detrimental impact on ecology.

Anthropocentrism supports and prioritises the exceptional status of the human within a whole earth community. The term human here represents human social, cultural and political systems that have standardised values and lifestyles at the expense of life that does not subscribe to this paradigm.

The latter might include the earth-based cultures that have been colonised, as well as life beyond the human sphere.

Assemblage is the gathering of multiple and contingent relationships that form a matrix of inquiry.

Attunement is the relational, empathic matching of communication that Massumi (2015) describes as 'the direct capture of attention and energies' (115) within a meeting place that brings an affective charge.

Becoming is the dynamic, relational transformation of material-discursive phenomena in the process of diversification. Becoming is a liminal, in-between, non-static process that refuses the definition of any particular state. It is a place of immanence.

Body is a conceptual notion that can be considered and experienced from many vertices, for example, physical, sensory, emotional, spiritual, environmental, cultural, social and political. Identity politics locates bodies within socio-political and cultural constructs such as race, gender, sexual orientation, disability and class. Bodies can be seen as 'permeable, moved by forces of affect and implicated in multisensory relations that constitute worlds' (Fullagar & Taylor, 2022: 39).

Bodying is a term used by Manning (2014), who proposes that '(a) philosophy of the body never begins with the body: it *bodies*' (163), preferring body as a verb (to body) rather than a noun (a body). This processual idea of what bodies do cuts across Cartesian binaries, as bodying processes affect and are affected within ecologies of movement.

Body without organs (BwO) is a philosophical conceptualisation of the notion of a body, troubling social, cultural and political inscriptions that become infused into our subjectivity at a visceral level. Deleuze and Guattari (1987) denote the complexity of bodies as social, political and cultural, philosophical and biological constructs.

Corporeality refers to moving bodies being created by, whilst also being the creators of, social, political and cultural identities.

Countertransference describes powerful inner states triggered in therapists through their interaction with clients. This happens in the less conscious realms of experience and is rich material within the relationship. Countertransference has the potential for relational exploration in service of the client, whilst also being an area that holds potential to provoke the therapists' acting out.

Dance is improvisational and/or choreographed corporeal participation in a world of material bodies.

Dance movement psychotherapy (DMP) is a psychotherapeutic intervention that recognises relational moving bodies as central and essential to the process. DMP is one of the arts therapies.

Data are the subjects and processes of research inquiry that gather into assemblages. From posthuman and new materialist perspectives, it is interesting to consider how and what data are privileged as well as how data emerge as entangled phenomena in relation to the researcher and the research process. Data are always situated and might be considered as events within assemblages.

Data that glow is a research term explored by Maclure (2013) denoting some fragment of datum that 'starts to glimmer, gathering our attention' (661) often on a sensory, intuitive and/or embodied level. It is data that find us, rather than data for which we go looking.

Decolonial attitudes acknowledge and resist the dominance of particular social, cultural and political power structures that have historically served to create hierarchical structures that disadvantage and exploit particular groups of people.

Deterritorialisation is a process of disruption that shifts the normativity inherent in belief systems and assumptions, for example, those underpinning binary oppositional pairs of dominating and subordinating hierarchies, to create new ways of thinking about and organising practices. Processes of deterritorialisation problematise territorialising forces of power relations. See Deleuze and Guattari (1987).

Diffraction is a term derived from quantum physics (Barad, 2007) and as a research methodology refers to the multiple possibilities of potential that are created in the convergence, divergence and collision of things. As a research methodology, diffraction supports the bringing together of disparate elements of multiple data, feeding them through and across each other and creating non-linear patterns of difference.

Disability is a category of social identity that denotes physical and/or cognitive differences identified in relation to normative benchmarks.

Discourse is an exchange of ideas through language. Critical discourses examine social, cultural and political power structures and constructs.

Ecofeminism is an immersion in a mutually implicated connectivity that challenges power differentials within gender politics, as it is entangled in intersectionality and environmental inequalities. Ecofeminists are not a homogenous group, and each individual who might identify as such will also bring a different way of inhabiting that identity.

Ecological self is a term originally coined by deep ecologist Naess (1995). It denotes a notion of selfhood that is embodied and embedded intra-dependently within a transversal ecological field; that is, the identity of the individual (the self) is mutually implicated within the identity of the ecology.

Ecopsychotherapy is an eclectic profession that brings an ecological lens to the practice of psychotherapy. It is aligned with the theories and practices of ecopsychology and ecotherapy and links individual psychological, emotional and psychic distress to the escalation of an environmentally destructive consumer culture in post-industrial capitalism that operates at the expense of the ecology.

Entanglement is the idea that material-discursive phenomena are always mutually implicated in some way. It is not possible to consider these phenomena in isolation of their entanglement without seeing each one as a part-object of some kind.

Epistemology is a philosophical theory of the nature of knowledge; that is, how do we know what we know and what it means to know? It is the parameters within which knowledge emerges.

Ethico-onto-epistemology is a neologism coined by Barad (2007) that conflates the terms ethics, ontology and epistemology. Barad refuses the division between ethics, ontology and epistemology as separate entities, claiming their entangled intra-action as an imperative.

Ethics refers to the ways in which equality and justice are thought about and applied.

Ethnography is the study of how particular cultures are lived out. Auto-ethnography is a research method that uses subjective experience to make sense of wider cultural phenomena, beliefs, and practices.

Holding environment is a term coined by Winnicott (1971) to describe the provision of good enough care that is psychologically, physically and emotionally safe and nourishing.

Humanism is a system of belief in a common humanity founded on rational and moral values and empathy for human beings and other sentient life.

Human exceptionalism is an anthropocentric notion referring to the human species as superior to and separate from other forms of life. This position then justifies environmental exploitation. Abram (1996) argues that the logic of species exceptionalism is also used to categorise some humans as 'not fully human' (48), but subordinating groups of people within a species hierarchy.

Kinaesthetic refers to the sensory, physical and emotional experience of moving bodies in space and time.

Kinship refers to an intimate relational connectivity that fosters a strong attachment. Posthumanism and ecopsychotherapy include kinship within a multispecies community of players. Fostering transversal kinship through, for example, environmental movement brings a focus to the intimacy of our relationships across species and landscapes.

Knowledge emerges in many guises. Posthuman and new materialist research inspire different ways of thinking about how knowledge is privileged and what determines that process of privileging.

Immanence is a concept at the heart of posthuman research as an ontological imperative. Immanence is about the connectivity and dynamic movement that is going on continuously an intra-subjective level.

Intersectionality is a term coined by Crenshaw (1991) to challenge feminist identity politics in that it failed to acknowledge the complexity of lived differences in its analysis of gender, particularly with regard to race. Whilst rooted in critical race theory, intersectionality can be applied to multiply marginalised social identities.

Intra-action is a neologism coined by Barad (2007) to represent the idea that phenomena continuously emerge from relational dynamics, rather than separate phenomena pre-existing that relationship. Intra-action is the relational connectivity of all matter.

Intra-subjectivity is the notion that subjectivity comprises entangled, relational phenomena that are mutually implicated in material-discursive processes.

Line of flight is a term to denote intra-active interruptions and disruptions that are non-linear and to some extent acausal. A line of flight leads to the new, the unanticipated and the unexpected. See Deleuze and Guattari (1987).

Managerialism is based on systems of management within organisations that are tightly controlled, predictable, top-down linear structures of defined goals and targets. A system of managerialism is characterised by hyper-rationality (Dalal, 2018)

Material-discursive is a hyphenated neologism referring to the mutually constituted nature of materiality (i.e., the physical presence of phenomena) and discourse (the representative thinking and critique linked to phenomena).

Neoliberalism is a political ideology that favours individualism and marketisation through deregulated economic and social systems.

Neologism is a newly created word, phrase and/or acronym, often evolving from an existing word or words that become a line of flight into new concepts and meanings, often bringing together multiple ideas.

New materialism is a precursor of posthumanism and provides a theoretical, interdisciplinary, socio-political field of inquiry that brings a focus to the significance of all matter as performative actors in an emergent, intra-active web of relations.

Ontology is the philosophy of being, that is, the nature of existing in the world: how we come to think about what things are, what exists and what is real. This is an interesting idea when applied to moving bodies and the transient nature of improvisational dance.

Other refers to the not-like-us who become marginalised and subordinated.

Performativity is the expression of social, cultural and political inscriptions that manifest as part of the identity politics of, for example, gender, race, disability and sexual orientation.

Postcolonialism is a discourse that critiques the dominance of social, cultural and political power structures that have created hierarchies. Postcolonialism creates a paradigm that refuses and challenges colonial discourses that have disadvantaged and exploited groups of peoples.

Postqualitative research resists mechanised research methodologies, emphasising the centrality of ethics, ontology and epistemology (ethico-onto-epistemology) that fosters multiplicity and works with material-discursive tensions and contradictions. See Murris (2021), Lather and St Pierre (2013) and St Pierre (2014).

Posthumanism moves beyond the humanist position, critiquing the social, political, environmental and species oppressions that have been inherent in the white, Eurocentric historical notion of what constitutes the idea of a human. Posthumanism challenges the notion of the human as an autonomous, independent subject that is not already implicated in a relational intra-active process.

Practice as research (PaR) refers to research methodologies that generate knowledge through practice.

Practivism is a form of practice that is an inherent act of resistance.

Queer theory refuses essentialism and the power-laden binary oppositions that arise from it, with particular reference to gender, sex and sexuality. To queer knowledge production is to challenge what belongs and what gets excluded.

Race is a social, cultural and political identity construction. It is one of the protected characteristics of the Equality Act 2010.

Rhizome is a metaphor that supports research and practice. The rhizome is a horizontal underground system of multiple roots and shoots arising from different places. Deleuze and Guattari (1987) used this metaphor of multiplicity, complexity and plurality to bring ideas together, with an emphasis on the flows between phenomena, rather than the phenomena themselves.

Site-specific refers to research and practice in which the location, either indoors or outdoors, is crucial to the process.

Spacetimemattering is a neologism created by Barad (2007) to denote the mutually implicated nature of space, time and matter, none of which can exist independently of the other, none of which occupies linearity and all of which are emergent.

Thing power theorises a kind of materiality in which all matter is entangled in a relational, energetic ecology, moving beyond a simple binary of human/non-human (Bennett, 2010).

Transference refers to the relational, dynamic processes between therapists and clients through which the past experience of significant relationships is projected into live interactions.

Transversality cuts across phenomena.

Worlding is an immersion in the world that finds diverse kinships.

References

Abram, D. (1996). *The Spell of the Sensuous*. New York: Vintage Books.

Barad, K. (2007). *Meeting the Universe Halfway: Quantum Physics and the Entanglement of Matter and Meaning*. London: Duke University Press.

Bennett, J. (2010). *Vibrant Matter: A Political Ecology of Things*. Durham: Duke University Press.

Crenshaw, K. (1991). Mapping the margins: Intersectionality, identity politics, and violence against women of color. *Stanford Law Review*, Vol. 43, No. 6, pp. 1241–1299.

Dalal, F. (2018). *The Cognitive Behavioural Tsunami: Managerialism, Politics and the Corruption of Science*. Oxon: Routledge.

Deleuze, G. and Guattari, F. (1987). *A Thousand Plateaus: Capitalism and Schizophrenia*. London: Continuum.

Fox, N. and Alldred, P. (2015). New materialist social inquiry: Designs, methods and the research-assemblage. *International Journal of Social Research Methodology*, Vol. 18, No. 4, pp. 399–414.

Fullagar, S. and Taylor, C. (2022). Body. In K. Murris (ed.), *A Glossary for Doing Postqualitative, New Materialist and Critical Posthumanist Research across Disciplines*, pp. 38–39. Oxon: Routledge.

Lather, P. and St. Pierre, E. (2013). Post-qualitative research. *International Journal of Qualitative Studies in Education*, Vol. 26, No. 6, pp. 629–633.

MacLure, M. (2013). Researching without representation? Language and materiality in post-qualitative methodology. *International Journal of Qualitative Studies in Education*, Vol. 26, No. 6, pp. 658–667.

Manning, E. (2014). Wondering the world directly – or, how movement outruns the subject. *Body and Society*, Vol. 20, Nos. 3–4, pp. 162–188.

Massumi, B. (2015). *The Politics of Affect*. Cambridge: Polity Press.

Murris, K. (ed.). (2021). Making kin: Postqualitative, new materialist and posthumanist research. In K. Murris (ed.), *Navigating the Postqualitative, New Materialist and Critical Posthumanist Terrain across Disciplines: An Introductory Guide*, pp. 1–21. Oxon: Routledge.

Naess, A. (1995). Self-realization: An ecological approach to being in the world. In G. Sessions (ed.), *Deep Ecology for the Twenty-First Century: Readings on the Philosophy and Practice of the New Environmentalism*, pp. 225–239. Boulder: Shambhala Publications.

St Pierre, E. (2014). A brief and personal history of post qualitative research toward "Post Inquiry". *Journal of Curriculum Theorizing*, Vol. 30, No. 2, pp. 2–19.

Winnicott, D. W. (1971). *Playing and Reality*. London: Tavistock.

Foreword

To read this book is to embark on an adventure, but not an adventure into distant, unknown exotic lands, rather into the unremarkable ordinary that has always been present but unnoticed, and to see it anew for the first time.

But the book is also an adventure into distant, unknown exotic lands – at least for this reader, ignorant of ecofeminism, posthumanism and new materialism. But paradoxically, it is these (to me) novel perspectives which bring the unremarkable (and unremarked) ordinary into view.

What is this kind of writing? Is it prose? Is it poetry? Surely it is both, surely it is more: sometimes it is a haiku:

> Breathing in, I unfold my spine and straighten my legs to stand upright, facing the world.
> Outside the window rain falls

Neophyte novelists are advised that they should not *tell* (he was angry), rather they should *show* (he shouted and smashed the glass). Wittgenstein speaks to something similar in saying that some things cannot be spoken of, they can only be shown. This is what Frizell does: she walks the talk, in that her way of writing is to inhabit, embody and even perform the world view and methodology she wants to put forward before us. The form and the content are congruent with each other. Frizell does not describe from 'outside,' rather she shows from the 'inside.' In this way, she privileges not only subjectivity but also the material.

The book is most remarkable for the attention to the mostly unnoticed detail that not only surrounds but also, and most importantly, *impacts* and *informs* the normalised accounts of the psychotherapy process. Frizell does not explain that this is so, but as ever she shows us that this is so.

Reading this work has made me realise how much it is that I do not notice and see because I must subliminally think it unimportant, as just so much noise. I think that I am noticing things, but clearly not enough! I am reminded of a tennis coach saying to a young player 'watch the ball' and the player replying, 'I am watching the ball,' to which she says 'watch the ball more!' Similarly, I need to develop my capacity to notice 'more.' When Frizell brings these elements to my attention, I come to realise what I took to be mute and inanimate actually speaks; all I need to do is learn how to listen.

It is somewhat humbling to witness the degree and detail of attention Frizell is able to bring not only to her client but also to the surrounding contexts which somehow matter to the work. I am reminded of the philosopher/activist/mystic Simone Weil saying that 'Those who are unhappy have no need for anything in this world but people capable of giving them their attention' (Weil, 1973 [1951]: 114). Frizell is certainly capable of paying attention and knowing it to be profound. Weil says, 'Attention is the rarest and purest form of generosity' (Weil, 1942: 18).

I discover that dead matter speaks. It is alive; more accurately, when Frizell brings it alive, it speaks.

The dark green satin lining of the coat catches the sun who is momentarily streaming through the window.

I finally understand this must be what new materialism is referring to.
I discover that the non-human world also speaks to clients and therapists.

We sit quietly for a minute or two. I remind myself that there is no rush as I listen to the delicacy of the moment. A blackbird's mellow song punctuates the edge of the silence.

As did the crow . . .
I finally understand this is what must be meant by the posthuman.

A warning reader: this is not going to be a passive read. Frizell will periodically jolt you into activity with what she calls 'provocations,' inviting you to become aware of your state of mind and emotional world as you read. And if that isn't enough, she will invite you to express these states through some creative activity, movement, song and the like. In this way, she will draw you into what she calls 'the materiality of the body, the freedom of creative process and the wisdom of less conscious worlds, as well as stimulating new perspectives through language and discourse.'

Frizell does not forget to attend to the social world, power differentials, processes of inclusion and exclusion, and so on. Her way of doing it is organic: she weaves in the personal, the political, the social, the psychological, the material, the crow, the stone and the look; and she does it seamlessly.

Be warned: the book will change your way of looking at things; indeed, things will no longer simply be 'things' – it did me.

Dr Farhad Dalal is a UK-based independent psychotherapist, group analyst and author.

Farhad Dalal

References

Weil, S. (1942). Letter to poet Joe Bousquet. In S. Pétriment (ed.), *Simone Weil: A Life*. New York: Schocken Books.
Weil, S. (1973). *Waiting on God*. New York: First Harper Colophon, 1951.

Prologue
Cliff moves

On the wild Tin Coast at Botallack on the south-west coast of England, disused mineshafts hold memories of thousands of tons of copper, tin and arsenic produced between 1815 and 1914. Lives of all kin(ds) were lost, and scars of plundering are etched into the rock. I peer into the entrance of a mineshaft to see broken train tracks disappearing into a dark, silent abyss. Further along the coast, the green metallic glow alludes to precious metals in the earth. The fierce easterly wind disturbs discarded litter and an empty packet of crisps blows out to the sea.

We continue along the coast to park at Zennor. Smartly dressed church-goers bow their heads against the wind on their way to St Senara's Sunday service. The church bells ring in the belfry that towers into a blue sky. Inside the church, a 600-year-old oak chair bears the carving of a mermaid who, sitting on a rock below Zennor, became mesmerised by the voice of a choir boy. She ventured closer and one Sunday enticed him down to the sea. Neither was seen again. This part-human, female seductress had lured a choir boy from his innocence in a story cautioning against the female other(ing).

Descending to the coastal path from Zennor, we begin the exhilarating walk. I clamber over rocks, ascending and descending the sometimes water-logged, sometimes steep and often winding path. I am danced by an elemental vitality amongst families of seals, diving gannets and a vast electrifying sea-scape. The wind leans into my back and hurries billowing clouds across the sky. The sun throws shadows across rolling waves, shifting the blueness from dark to light and all shades in between.

With one headland accomplished, another looms and another and yet another and eventually I turn a corner to see St Ives, flanked by golden beaches. Arriving into the town, I pass the Tate St Ives gallery and chance upon an exhibition entitled *From Where I Stand* (Nkanga, 2019) by the performance artist Otobong Nkanga, whose work enlivens ideas about bodies, landscapes and multiple ways of being here together. Tapestries, photos, paintings and objects investigate the human propensity for compulsive consumption of the earth's natural resources. An enormous tapestry entitled 'The weight of scars' (ibid) combines textiles and photography illustrating (headless) figures grasping at ropes connected to more ropes, pipelines and pictures of abandoned

DOI: 10.4324/9781003322658-1

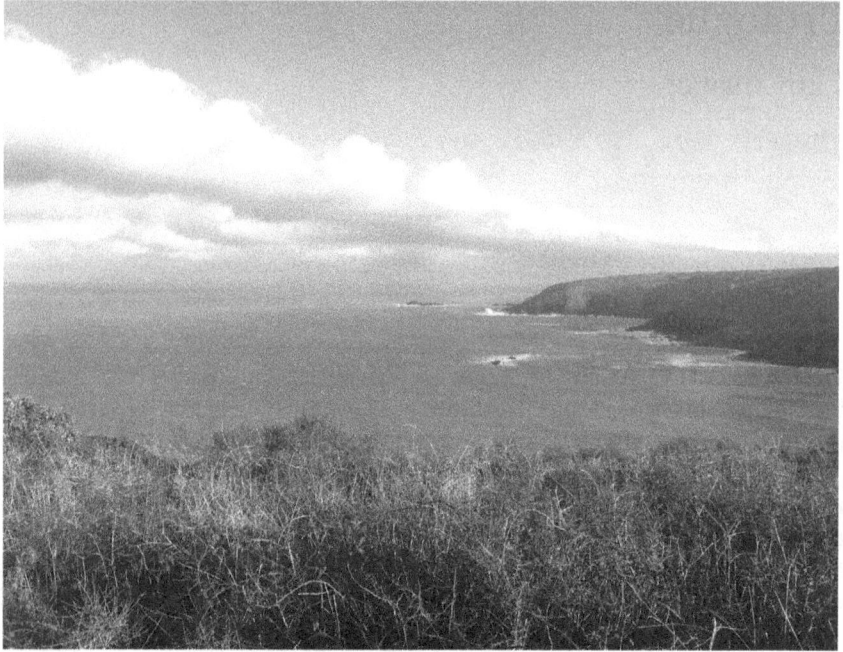

Figure 0.1 Zennor to St Ives.
Source: Photograph by author.

mineshafts. The pushing and pulling of multiple arms inflict a violence on the earth that unsettles my spirit.

****

This book calls for a gentle strength that enables us to move through the world softly, respectfully and with lightness of foot towards ecofeminist, post-human possibilities.

Reference

Nkanga, O. (2019). Imagining the scars of a landscape. *Tate*. *YouTube*. https://youtube/qZZruEToDCI

1 Becoming

Outside the kitchen window, a green woodpecker alights on the grass. She[1] zig-zags across the lawn before swooping away with a yaffle that makes me smile. I wander into the garden with my mug of tea. The fluted call of a song thrush threads through the morning like a silk ribbon from the topmost branch of a silver birch. I shiver in the crisp breeze that cuts through the April sun. Daffodils are coming to an end and trees are budding with potential. Yellow primroses sit at the foot of the magnolia and wispy clouds scud in the wind. The swallows have not arrived yet, I think, as I settle on the blue garden bench. I contemplate Maeve, the new client who will be arriving in a few moments. I place my elbows on my knees and cup my hands around my mug of tea, threading my middle fingers through the outward facing handle to enjoy its warmth in the palms of my hands. My mind replays our email exchange. It took a while to firm up a consultation time as Maeve was uncertain if she could make any of my available dates. A bulbous beetle topples over blades of grass at my feet, her blue-black back glinting in the sun. I take my mug back to the kitchen and go into the studio, noticing a charged feeling in my chest. I sit, feeling awkward, and shift position. As the clock confirms one minute before our agreed time, I hear the underside of the wooden door slide across the thick carpet tiles. I walk across the studio to the half open door. A crow squawks outside the window. A woman in her early 50s looks directly at me. She is wearing a brown herringbone wool coat, buttoned up to the neck. Maeve is slightly older than I imagined. I smile, noticing my head tilting to the right with curiosity. A crow squawks – this time from a distance.

'Hello, you must be Maeve.'

Maeve laughs nervously and takes a step back as she fumbles to undo the top button of her coat. At the second button, she turns to look at

DOI: 10.4324/9781003322658-2

the upright chair beside her and then looks back at me, stepping forward to bring her feet together.

'You can leave your coat and shoes out here.'

I grasp the studio door handle and stand awkwardly across the threshold, like a beetle tumbling through the grass.

'Yes, sure,' she says, continuing to unbutton her coat and the dark green satin lining catches the sun that momentarily streams through the window.

Maeve folds her coat neatly with the lining outside and drapes it carefully across the cushioned seat of the upright chair. The sun highlights a cobweb on the shelf above. She holds onto the back of the chair and uses the toe of her right foot to lever off one boot, which she shakes to the floor before resting her right foot across her left knee to pull off the other. Placing her boots side by side under the chair, she follows me through the door without making a sound. The door is slightly stiff as the oak wood has expanded in the damp weather. I push hard to close it and we recalibrate momentarily after the punctuated bang of the door. Maeve looks around the room and I look at Maeve, lifting my arm to indicate the two chairs at the other end of the studio. Her small, quick steps contrast the rhythm of my own stride. I feel big and clumsy. Sitting down, Maeve runs both hands simultaneously down the red velvet arms of her chair. Repeating the movement, she looks from one hand to the other with a look of delight. With her hands still in contact with the chair cover, she looks at me and takes a deep breath in.

'I love the feel of this chair,' she says.

I feel a warm glow of pride for these chairs that I came across by chance in a small shop in Penzance some time before. Maeve is now brushing the material back and forth with the back of her right hand, and the red velvet darkens and lightens in response.

'Would you look at that softness,' she says, with a rising intonation.

I smile, touched by Maeve's sensory delight in the material cover of the chair. I am drawn to her soft lilting accent, not unlike that of my long-gone maternal grandmother.

We sit quietly for a minute or two. I remind myself that there is no rush as I listen to the delicacy of the moment.

A blackbird's mellow song punctuates the edge of the silence.

Becoming entangled

As I welcomed Maeve[2] into the studio, we were already mutually implicated in an entanglement that began as we entered the orbit of each other's awareness. In my account of Maeve's arrival, I bring attention to some of the multiple unfoldings of the world in any one moment. In anticipation of Maeve's arrival, I spent a few moments in the garden, resourcing myself with a cup of tea and a moment of reflection, locating myself in the materiality of my immediate world. Maeve and I were entering the unfolding of new potential in our work together and this vignette brings a sprinkling of just some of the intra-acting[3] participants within the emergent assemblage[4] of this becoming:

green woodpecker   mug of tea   song thrush   silver birch

crisp breeze   April sun   wilting daffodils   primroses

magnolia tree   wispy clouds   yet-to-arrive swallows

garden bench   beetle   blades of grass   kitchen   studio

clock   wooden door   thick carpet tiles   crow   window

herringbone coat   green satin lining   upright chairs   cobweb

pair of boots   floor   red velvet chair covers   blackbird

Each of these elements flowed in a relational field within my awareness and as part of a collective embodied embedment, in an unfolding world.

Becoming unfolding experiential worlds

This book explores how practice and research can move through such intra-active unfoldings as part of the poetry of experiential worlds. As the narrative of this book unfolds, I invite you to join me in the exploration of ecofeminist dance movement psychotherapy (DMP) research and practice, imagining what they can do, rather than what they are. I use the term ecofeminism to denote a practice principle of immersion in mutually implicated connections that challenge power differentials within gender politics and, at the same time, engage with entanglements of intersectional and environmental inequalities of these power differentials. We (those identifying as ecofeminists) will each explain, think about, implement and activate these principles differently and ecofeminism is a process that signposts multiple ways of becoming.[5] We are all moving through this territory differently. As I continue to move through ecofeminist landscapes, I have become aligned with the spirit of posthuman and new materialist perspectives and, in so doing, move away from positivist ideas about essentialism (i.e., defining the essence of predetermined entities) towards ideas that are creative and processual (i.e., constantly in the emergent process of evolving, creating and being created). This immanence is a place of becoming. It is embedded in the corporeality of spontaneous and indeterminate moving bodies (of all kin(ds)), along with wider social, cultural, political and environmental discourses that are implicit in that corporeality. It refuses notions of single truths that await discovery and engages with eco-ethical participation in the intra-active ecology of the world. Posthuman and new materialist perspectives that underpin this approach will be explained in more detail in subsequent chapters, specifically Chapter 2.

Each chapter of this book begins with a vignette from the therapeutic relationship that evolves between Maeve and me. Rather than presenting a chronological description of the process, I have selected vignettes that sketch non-linear, thematic grains in which I track my own process as practitioner-researcher and researcher-practitioner as it became entangled in this intervention.

This initial meeting with Maeve came about when she responded to my callout for participants in a case study research inquiry that comprised individual DMP sessions for 40 weeks. After replying to her initial email, I heard nothing back for a while and just as I was assuming it was one of those inquiries that might not materialise, Maeve responded. This ambivalence manifested during the process and was rich material for exploration. In this initial meeting, we began to think together about the possibility of Maeve's participation in a practice-led case study inquiry into the processes of psychodynamic DMP through an ecofeminist lens of new materialism and posthumanism.[6] It was also an initial consultation to think about the possibility of Maeve and I working together as therapist and client within this research context. The complexities of that decision, along with ethical issues of consent, will be unpacked in Chapter 6, which focuses on the research.

And for now, I wonder how you are arriving into this first chapter. I wonder how you came across this book. I wonder where you imagine that it will take you. I wonder if you are reading a paper hard copy or an online copy and the story behind that choice. I wonder where you are in terms of the materiality of your immediate location as you read. Here is a suggested provocation for you to begin to create your own part in this dialogic process of reading this book:

Take a moment to notice how entering this book is situated for you. How you are arriving? What are the lenses that you are bringing to this process through your practising, theorising and researching and/or through your lived experience.

I invite you to map out this assemblage through improvised dance, artwork, music, roleplay and/or in free-flow writing.

Such provocations will be woven through the narrative of this book, more generally at the end of each chapter, to invite you as an active agent into the materialisation of these ideas. These provocations invite a creative, dialogic process as we (you and I) enter into the sometimes familiar and sometimes unfamiliar, always with possibilities of moving through alternative vertices, bringing

embodied creativity into the heart of innovative research, methodological frameworks for practice and practice-in-its-very-becoming.

(Frizell & Rova, 2023: 1)

These invitations through creative experiential provocations aim to bring you home into the materiality of the body, the freedom of creative process and the wisdom of less conscious worlds, as well as stimulating new perspectives through language and discourse.

Becoming present

Therapy is a very private affair, yet the personal is always political. When we begin to explore the connecting threads between individual and organisational well-being, the health of social, political and economic structures and the health of the planet, it would be incomplete to consider any one of these things in isolation. Maeve's engagement with therapy was no exception. The first few sessions with Maeve served as an assessment that offered us both opportunities to think about the possibility of working together in the therapeutic process and as part of a research project, including the necessary risk assessments and the potential compatibility of what I offered as well as what Maeve wanted and needed. Throughout the process, we continued to arrive into new possibilities, as we explored multiple narratives that were colliding with and shaping the ways that Maeve lived her life.

As I am imagining you reading this book, perhaps you could imagine me sitting here at the computer, struggling with how to arrive (repeatedly) into this writing, making decisions about which words go where, as I feel my way into the different possibilities of articulating ecofeminist research and practice with differently moving bodies as a modality of focus. I sit at a desk festooned with books and printed articles, new and old, always hoping that they might provide an answer. To my left, a coffee cup and to my right, a purple pencil case oozing the optimism of freshers' week. A pot of hand cream is just within reach and the very thought of opening the lid to brush my fingertip across the surface of the thick aromatic cream and to spread it over the surface of both hands s-l-o-w-s me down, creating an interruption from the relentless online demands of the computer screen and bringing me back to the sensing moving body. The small sketch pad and a box of broken oil pastels with not-yet-made-it-to-the-bin picked-off paper covers remind me to move into colour, shape and an externalised image. And behind my chair is a small space to move, inviting me to shift away from the screen and immerse myself in the experience of the improvisational moving body.

I take the invitation, shifting the three books that have already intruded on that floorspace.

I swing my legs around to the side of the chair, stand up and face away from my desk. With my feet comfortably apart, my knees bend, I curve my spine and rest my hands lightly on my thighs. My shoulders drop, and I lower my head, feeling a gentle stretch as my neck takes the weight of my head. My hands brush over my knees and out into the space. As I lift my head, I catch sight of the world. I feel alone as the cream-coloured wall looks back at me. I catch my weight on my right foot and sweep my left arm across my body, to follow a wide sweeping motion that moves rhythmically from the right to the left, to the right, to the left through a fluid, sequential motion, like a boat rocking gently on silver water. The momentum falls away and returning to the centre ground, I bring both arms in towards my chest and push the air in front of me as my knees soften into a bend and my spine pushes backwards. I hold the curve for a moment. Breathing in, I unfurl my spine and straighten my legs to stand upright, facing the world.

Outside the window, rain falls.

Returning to my desk, I look out of the window at the laurel bush, behind which is a streetlamp where a pair of blue tits made their nest last spring and the spring before that. To one side of the streetlamp, a wisteria yields to the rain.

The stories of this world of things are multiple.

Becoming material through the power of things

I sit here aware of my relational proximity to all these material things involved in the immediate unfolding of this writing. Ahmed (2010) points out that an orientation towards writing involves a range of material things that enable that writing to happen and those things all have stories of significance. For example, this desk at which I sit would have been something that my grandmother would have cleaned to enable (more likely than not) a man to write, as a working-class woman born in 1897. And now, I claim this desk to write as a political act (ibid) and as I do so, I identify as a parent-carer-scholar-practitioner-researcher-therapist-educator. As I reflect on how I am immediately situated, I become conscious of the '(t)hing power' (Bennett, 2010: 20) of which I am a part, through orientations that are both personal and political.

This *thing power* was brought to my attention by my youngest daughter when moving from the family home in north London. We were leaving a community that we had come to value as our three children had grown up. I had anticipated missing the neighbours, the local park, the nearby café, the garden, the frog spawn in the pond and the hedgehog snuffling across the lawn by the light of the moon. However, my daughter brought my attention to small details in the house, to which she had an attachment: a small chip in the skirting board that resembled a fish, the slightly battered metal Edwardian bedroom doorknob, the green plastic crocodile that had been stuffed down the back of the bathroom radiator during a sibling squabble, the tessellated tiles on the hallway floor and the Christmas card written in French, trapped between two floorboards under the carpet. In a re-membering ritual, she took photos of material details that had been part of her becoming, foregrounding the thing power that Bennet (2010) suggests is

> a good starting point for thinking beyond the life-matter binary, the dominant organizational principle of adult experience.
>
> (20)

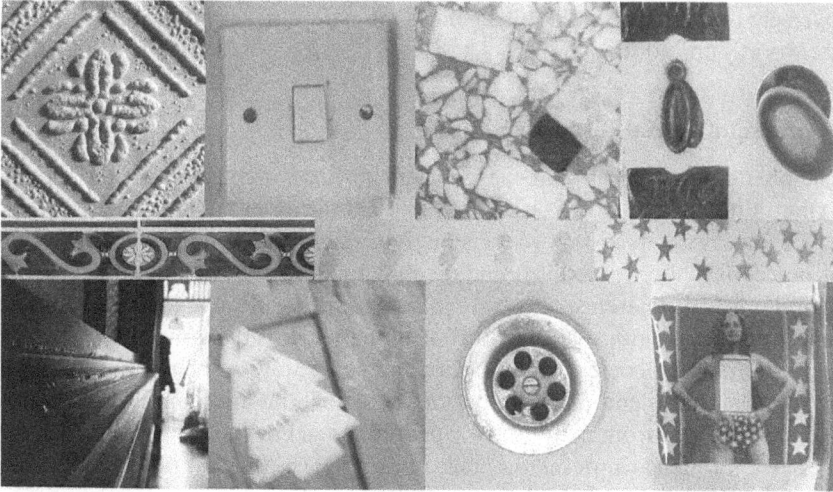

Figure 1.1 Material things.
Source: Compilation of photographs by the author's daughter.

I found myself re-membering the wonder in small things through the eyes of a child, listening out for small things as knowledge-ing messengers. Taylor (2021) uses the term 'knowledge-ing' (28) (as a verb, rather than a noun) to denote knowledge as a shifting, fluid process that is part of bigger, wider, longer and deeper happenings that are always going on.

Becoming knowledge(ing)

This book commits to a kind of knowledge-making that challenges how some *things* (and by *things*, I refer to the material and the discursive) become privileged over others. For example, in Western education systems, intellect, language and discourse are privileged over the emotional, sensory, material and experiential integrity of being in the world. The things that get to count as knowledge are inscribed with particular social, political, economic, cultural and environmental notions of privilege and entitlement. New materialist and posthuman voices (human and otherwise) of ecofeminism trouble the notion of how things come to matter and how knowledge is privileged, unsettling the human-centred perspectives (perhaps more specifically, particular-kinds-of-human-centred) of the anthropocene.[7] Through this writing, I invite you to explore ecofeminist, new materialist and posthuman possibilities of researching and practising that lean towards

> the corporeal matter of the practice of knowledge-ing that is grounded in doing and becoming, rather than in defining and being.
>
> (Frizell, 2023a: 66)

As you read this book, I invite you to stay with the trouble (Haraway, 2016) as diversely (dis)enabled, relational bodies animate different possibilities within the world's unfolding.

Becoming material-discursive bodies

The phenomenological philosopher Merleau-Ponty (2004) reminded us that '(t)he things of the world are not simply neutral objects which stand before us for our contemplation' (48), encouraging our attention towards the world of perception. Posthumanism and new materialism widen this phenomenological frame of reference, fostering ideas about the affective capacity (i.e., the capacity to affect and to be affected) of all matter. It is this privileging of some matter(s) (some peoples, some species and some ways of being in the world) over others that is embedded in pervasive inequalities and oppressions.

I have learned from many autistic people the richness of bringing a focus to the small moment-to-moment details of experience. I have worked with many clients and participants who have no spoken words with which to relate to the world. The realms of communication beyond language, such as the sensory and emotional dimensions of material bodies in motion, become the place of arrival, of encounter, of relationship, of experience and of separation. That is, bodies *become*, again and again, through moving.

I remember an initial meeting with 11-year-old Jake who had recently arrived in the autistic unit of a special school in an urban inner-city environment. Just before meeting Jake, a member of his classroom staff team told me of his unpredictable tantrums in which he might self-harm or lash out at his environment. Rolling up her sleeve, she showed me a line of red scratch marks on her skin and in addition, she advised 'mind your hair.' I found my body bracing defensively at her words. Here, I describe my initial encounter with Jake.

Entering the classroom, I am struck by Jake's tall, lithe figure. I sense his alertness and sensitivity, although he makes no outward sign of being aware of my presence. Jake stands at the side of the room, shifting his weight from one foot to another. His focus is on his right index finger curling and uncurling with clockwork precision a few inches from his face. Jake begins to rock rhythmically in time with his finger.

I greet the other two young people in the room, noticing that I find comfort in my familiarity with their rituals and reminding myself how unfamiliar they too had both seemed when I had first met them. Moving slowly, I sit at a spare desk, intuiting that being seated might make me seem less of a threat. Jake's finger stops moving and he punctuates his flow with a sharp turn of the head, tilting one side of his face up to the corner of the room, seemingly mirroring my spatial shift. With a lurch that takes me by surprise, he runs around the edge of the room, passing behind me and burying himself in the crevasse between a large blue beanbag and the wall. He remains there for what seems like a long time. I find my attention wandering and I begin to feel restless, noticing that Jake is disappearing from my awareness. I consciously bring my attention back and at this point, Jake emerges from behind the beanbag, placing it to one side and pulling his body along the floor to sit opposite me with his back against the wall, knees bent. He contorts his long fingers into a kaleido-scope of complex shapes in front of his eyes. I wonder if he is looking at me through his fingers.

I remain seated at my table, conscious not to look directly at him, but keeping him within the orbit of my vision, wondering if he is doing the same with me. His hands drop nonchalantly on to his legs and supporting his wrists on his knees, he begins to lift his fingers towards the ceiling before letting them flop downwards. As he repeats this action, he turns his head to look around the room. Our eyes meet momentarily. The brief intense glance signals to me that we have met.

Very slowly I stand up, walk around the edge of the room and settle on the floor against the wall a couple of metres away from Jake, bending my legs and resting my wrists over my knees. We turn our heads to look at each other, and I mirror the lifting and dropping of the fingers with my wrists supported on my knees. Jake has a look of curiosity on his face.

'Hello, Jake. I'm Caroline.'

He drops his hands down onto the floor with a thud that makes me jump and I lower my hands gently down to the same position. We continued to look at each other and his fingers drum the floor, making a light, rhythmic sound like falling rain. I listen carefully, sensing that it would be intrusive to join in. Jake's tapping slows to an even beat and we look at each other. I can hear my own breathing and I feel the solid wall against my spine. For a few moments, I am surprised to find that Jake's tapping and my heartbeat are synchronised. Jake turns his back on me and dives back into his hiding place under the bean bag. I slowly get up and make my way back to my seat at the table.

Without warning Jake springs to his feet and looks at an empty table expectantly. For a moment I am confused, until, within a few seconds of his jumping up, snack time is announced and a teaching assistant brings juice and biscuits to place them on the table.

As I recall that initial encounter, I'm reminded how my relationship with Jake was characterised by arriving into fragile, fleeting moments of relational connection that were mediated through the kinaesthetic sense of our moving bodies, rather than language. There was no linear path, however, together we moved into an understanding of the intra-connected relational space between us. This vignette illustrates how I created a responsive listening space, resisting the urge to frame, to shape, to formulate and to understand. I needed to im-merse myself in the materiality of the moment and to yield to the immersive experience that was unfolding in those improvisational, contingent turning places through which new possibilities emerged.

Becoming turning places

I have a photograph of myself from the early 1990s dancing at a Mayday celebration and in the picture, I am suspended in a place of transition, in the act of transferring my weight from one foot to another. The twist in my spine suggests an in-between-mo(ve)ment-of-potential, between two points of balance, teetering on the cusp of the past and future, happening, 'always and already in between' (Braidotti, 1997: 68), in a place that is 'relational, conjunctive and dynamic' (ibid).

This contingent place of becoming hovers in those in-between places . . .

. . . and . . .   . . . but . . .   . . . if . . .

. . . for . . .   . . . so . . .

. . . however . . .

. . . those links between one thought and another, one intention and another, one action and another. There is always the potential of turning towards becoming differently and of re-imagining and reconfiguring what we thought we knew. In this way, we are always arriving.

In creating this book, I remain open to those turning places that enable me to arrive and to arrive again, each time open to new potential. I write as an insider who is immersed in ecofeminist, new materialist, posthuman research and practice that embraces the diffractive meeting points of differently abled, differently situated and differently inscribed bodies.

Becoming situated

This book is (as all books are) situated: situated in my skills and experience as a practitioner and researcher; situated in a particular professional climate; situated in socio-political, economic and cultural landscapes and situated within an escalating ecological crisis. These chapters present an assemblage of my learning from professional practising, researching and lived experience that traversed the millennium into the first two decades of the twenty-first century.

The process of constructing this book has been rhizomatic, that is, a non-linear configuration that has multiple connections. Deleuze and Guattari (1987) present the rhizome as a root system metaphor that, rather than tracing back to a single source, arises from multiple sources. The authors point out that

any point of a rhizome can be connected to anything other, and must be. (7)

This rhizomatic, underground plant stem grows horizontally, creating a system of roots and shoots, in a non-linear configuration that holds the complexity of multiple points of convergence and emergence. An example of the astonishing potential of actual (rather than metaphoric) rhizomes can be found in Shark Bay, just off Australia's west coast. About 4,500 years ago, a single seed that had spawned from two different seagrass species found itself nestled in a favourable spot, and it has now grown into (probably) the biggest plant anywhere on Earth, covering an area equivalent to 20,000 football fields. The plant has spread using rhizomes and by sending out runners and continues to provide habitats for a huge array of marine species, including turtles, dolphins, dugongs, crabs and fish (Readfern, 2022).

Grounding my researching and practising in horizontal rhizomatic systems of moving, creating and thinking from multiple points of convergence and emergence offers the potential to shift away from the singularity of the vertical plane into the relationality of the horizontal plane. This writing draws on multiple points of emergence from 40 years' experience as a dance practitioner, dance movement psychotherapist, disability activist, author, senior lecturer and researcher, alongside the experience of the vicissitudes of everyday life, including raising three girls, now women, one of whom is learning-disabled and caring for elderly parents, providing end-of-life care and mourning their loss. In addition, I have drawn on my own personal process, including a decade of intensive Jungian analysis that included working outside in ancient woodland.

Becoming planted

The seeds of this book were sown when I decided to bring together a decade of research by engaging in writing a thesis for a PhD by publication. I happened to begin the thesis write-up just a few months before the COVID-19 global pandemic struck. Not only were my three children now grown up and living their own lives, but when the pandemic arrived, my work also either took place electronically or was cancelled. Lockdown put a stop to getting out and about for either work or play. I thus spent many hours at home developing a thesis that comprised a critical commentary of selected published research of my own carried out across more than 10 years. At the start of the PhD by publication, I found myself moving away from the more traditional qualitative research methods that I had used in previous research and moving towards new materialist and posthuman thinking. I was conscious that

(t)he methods we use as researchers are only as potent as the kind of thinking we use to think about those methods.

(Frizell, 2023b: 51–52)

That thesis was a launch pad for these chapters. However, creating a book from a thesis is a whole new diffractive turning point. After having the proposal for the publication accepted, I then needed to find some space to do what I am doing now (finalising the manuscript). I thus created a stretch of time, being granted dedicated research leave from my role as senior lecturer at Goldsmiths, University of London (thank you Goldsmiths), for 4 months and suspending my private practice of clients and supervisees (thank you to each one of you for your understanding) for this fixed period so that I could immerse myself in the writing. The finalising of the manuscript was inter-rupted by my father becoming ill and sadly dying and the publishers kindly extending my deadline.

On the first day of an intensive period of writing, I felt enormous gratitude for this writing space and reminded myself to keep in touch with creative pro-cesses, continuing to dance, create art, mould clay, play in the garden, go out for walks, dream and arrange play dates with colleagues, alongside sitting in front of a screen and putting words together. I wanted to be sure that ways of know-ing the world other than language were an integral part of this writing process.

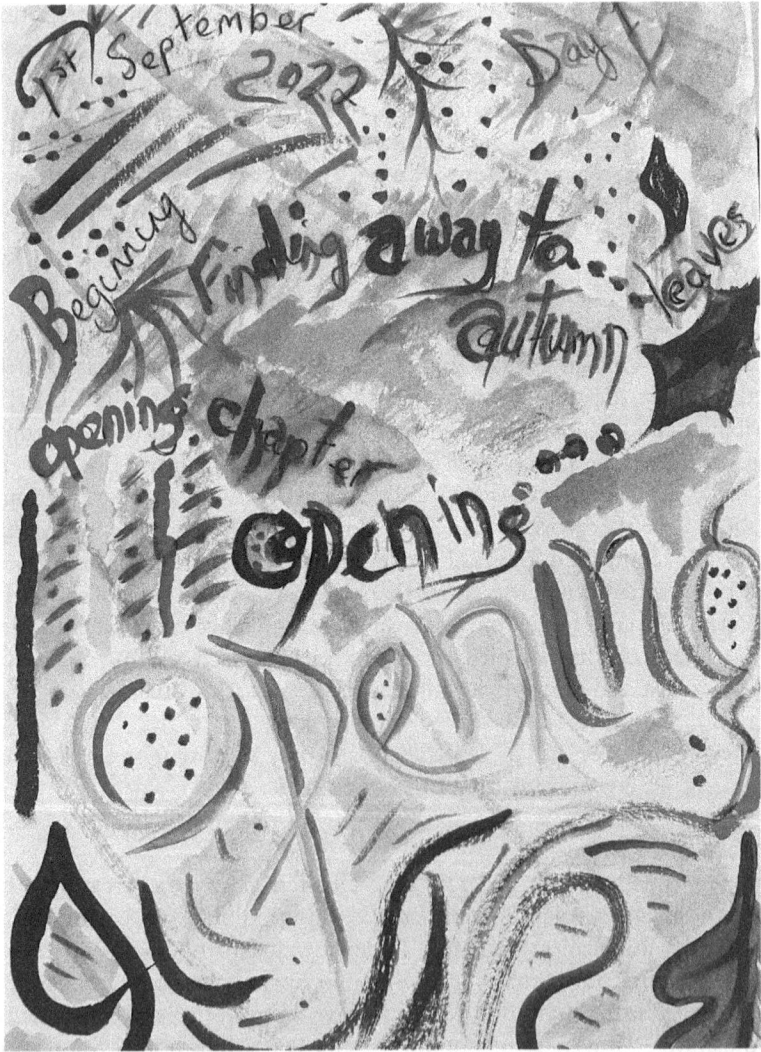

Figure 1.2 Opening.

Source: Photograph of a freehand doodle by the author.

That same day, I wandered into the garden and gathered some vegetables for a pasta sauce. I pulled a small red onion from the ground, picked four lush red tomatoes and three small shiny courgettes and cut some chard, with green and red stems. There had been little rain this summer and record temperatures had dried out much of the land. Some of the vegetables had been ruined due to the unusually hot dry weather and this was a clear and immediate reminder of the reality of the climate emergency. On my way to the kitchen, I took a garlic bulb from the braid of garlic that I had made when the crop was harvested. I found some music and before getting to work on the pasta sauce, I found myself moving across the kitchen floor, my arms opening out and my knees catching each step with a smooth sinking movement. Tentatively, I stepped forwards, not knowing where the movement was taking me. I was stepping into something new. I found myself acutely aware of being alone, yearning for a circle of fellow dancers to join me, with hands on each other's shoulders, to repeat step patterns rhythmically together, moving collectively as one body to the left and to the right. Putting dinner off even longer, I got out some watercolours and began to create a visual image. Some words soon began to blend into shapes, I seemed to be finding a way to navigate this opening chapter. The page was as colourful and as textured as the ingredients for the pasta sauce, freshly picked from the earth and now sitting on the kitchen worktop. I stepped back, to be struck by the word *opening*, and I reflected on this opening as an arrival and in that arrival, opening to ways of inhabiting this world that are

responsible and responsive to the world's patternings and murmurings.
(Barad, 2012: 207)

I washed my hands and made my way back to preparing the pasta sauce, offering apologies to my partner that dinner was going to be late!

As I was arriving into this writing, I was becoming situated as a practitioner, researcher, author, educator, mother, carer, (cook) and other identities within the ebb and flow of a relational world that is always in process. It is in that spirit that I offer you these chapters.

Becoming discursive

At the time of this book evolving, the world had recently been through the COVID-19 pandemic, which took hold globally in 2020, unfolding in a wave of loss and despair in all areas of life. At around this time, many inequalities of opportunity, of education, of health and of wealth that previously lurked unseen beneath media headlines had risen to the surface, some just prior to the pandemic and some amplified by the pandemic. The #MeToo movement brought protestation against a culture of sexual abuse, sexual harassment and the rape of women. The voice of the Black Lives Matter (BLM) movement called out racial discrimination, violence and inequalities following the murder of George Floyd at the hands of a police officer in 2020. Revelations about the institutional sexual abuse of disabled children, young people and adults by a celebrity in a position of power[8] who wilfully and freely abused these individuals for years, remaining unchallenged due to his celebrity status and abundant charity work. Environmental consciousness regarding ecological crisis had been catapulted into the mainstream arena, brought to our attention by wildfires, floods, desecration of communities and a rapid decline in biodiversity. The COVID-19 pandemic arrived on the back of long-term austerity measures in the UK, along with an escalation of neoliberal values, a referendum for the UK to leave the European Union and a landslide victory for right-wing politics. Social and political unrest made for continuous headline news, and entangled in that unrest was the urgency of the ecological crisis as it escalated, manifesting in disasters for living communities across the ecological web of life.

The need for social, political and environmental justice seemed more important than ever and this turbulent context was a provocation for me to orient my thinking differently about how identities are organised and how subjectivities are performed, in order to re-orient myself towards a more embodied, compassionate and empathic presence with the world. Public, political, academic and environmental discourses were moving towards a paradigm shift in response to rapid changes in the way we live our lives. This book moves with that tide, seeking to consider how creative, ecologically aware therapeutic practising and researching can be part of a gentle and powerful activism that refuses and resists oppressions that have become normalised, with injustices embedded in our everyday lives as well as in wider institutional and socio-politically governing systems. An ecofeminist approach, informed by posthumanism and new materialism, offers opportunities to move through orientations that refuse, resist and challenge how matter(s) come(s) to matter.

Becoming oriented

The chapters and interruptions in this book provide points of orientation through ethics (the application of justice), ontologies (ideas about *how* we exist in the world) and epistemologies (the nature of knowledge, as in what is known and how it is known). For some of you, particularly those who have engaged in research, those words *ethics, ontology* and *epistemology* might be familiar and comfortable. As for others, I expect you might gloss over the sentence or even begin to feel that this book isn't for you. But again, I remind you of my invitation to stay with trouble (Haraway, 2016). In fact, one of the threads that runs through this book *is* the very problem of the representational and abstract nature of language, along with an appreciation of language as part of a thinking apparatus that can help challenge deeply embedded social, political, cultural and environmental injustices. Barad (2003) reminds us how the dominance of language as a verbal modality is a bit of a sticking point, stating that

> (l)anguage has been granted too much power. The linguistic turn, the semiotic turn, the interpretative turn, the cultural turn: it seems that at every turn lately every 'thing' – even materiality – is turned into a matter of language or some other form of cultural representation.
>
> (801)

It is a struggle to hold on to the tension between the potential of language and discourse to help us better understand the world, language as a representation of experience (rather than the experience itself) and expressions of existences alternative to language, for example, through expressive modalities of dance, art, music, poetry and living experiences of all kin(ds).

Ecofeminist, new materialist and posthuman perspectives offer ways of thinking about the world (and by implication our work as practitioners, re-searchers and educators) that keep this struggle alive and bring our awareness to hierarchies of privilege, particularly regarding the phenomenon of power being granted disproportionately to language. The orientating principles of this book-as-an-assemblages-of-diverse-things are immersed in processes that shapeshift through moving bodies, rather than concepts to be entrapped by definitions. As these fluid processes move through points of convergence in this book-as-an-assemblage-of-diverse-things, I have found myself needing to draw on different genres of writing to bring to light the texture of ecofeminist researching and practising within a rapidly changing twenty-first century.

Becoming (in)conclusively

Throughout the book, I intentionally shift from the poetic to the prosaic, traversing different genres through story, poetry, critical commentary, imagin-ings and academic discourse. I ask you, the reader, to join me in this process of knowledge-ing (i.e., the process of generating knowledge) troubling the kinds of knowledge that is privileged (and indeed that might even be considered knowledge at all) and challenging how it is that some things, some people, some ideas and some modes of expression have come to matter more than others.

I invite you into some of the entanglements and contradictions that I have encountered as an ecofeminist DMP and movement artist, a research-led practitioner, a practice-led researcher and an educator in higher education in-stitutions, who immerses those practices in new materialist and posthuman processes. In order to stay with the trouble of *this* book as an assemblage, I hope that the structure enables you to orient yourself to experiential writing that weaves through the fabric of relevant theoretical and research scaffolding. The thematic chapters are punctuated with interruptions within a meandering stream of narratives that build intra-active, rhizomatic connections along the way. As you engage with the entanglements within this writing, you might read this book from cover to cover or you might flick through the pages, stopping at random moments when something resonates with you. You might just keep the book as a point of reference as you sharpen your own capacity for creative researching, writing and practising. You might fill the book with post-it notes, or doodle in the margins, as your own thoughts flow into new tributaries and/or change the current. Or, this might be one of those books that once purchased gets shifted from one bookshelf to another without get-ting read, yet remains alive (under the dust) as a potential in the fantasy that one day we will get through all that reading that is put aside for a later date! Whatever the diverse ways that you create a relationship with this book, I hope it provides a resource for researching and practising that honours and the in-separability of differentiating moving bodies of all kin(ds).

As I will discuss in later chapters, the professional practices entangled in the content of this book, that is, ecofeminist DMP and ecopsychotherapy, are, by nature, interdisciplinary and transdisciplinary, arising through the convergences of multiple practisings. These practisings are grounded in psychotherapeutic paradigms that converge with dance, movement and somatic practices for ecofeminist DMP and converge with deep ecology and environmental activism for ecopsychotherapy. The book creates a rhizomatic assemblage through transdisciplinary practices, drawing on issues of equality, diversity and inclusion, with particular (but not exclusive) reference to critical disability studies in order to deepen notions of the many ways that human subjectivity can manifest in a complex, intra-connected world. The book moves with a tide that is fostering a paradigm shift that seeks to challenge existing narratives through critical awareness and prioritises *caring* as an underlying principle for the health and well-being of the planet as a community.

As I bring this chapter to a close, I will take you back into the studio in which Maeve has arrived.

> As the blackbird's song punctuates the silence, Maeve takes her hands off the arms of the chair and put her clasped hands in her lap. She looks towards me with what I perceive as anxiety in her eyes.
>
> 'Well,' I say, 'here we are.'
>
> I smile and shift my weight slightly further back into my chair. I rest my hands in my lap and cross my left leg over my right.
>
> 'Perhaps you'd like to tell me a little about what has brought you here.'

And that is where this book begins. As you and I arrive into this unfolding, I invite you to think about your own arrival through the following provocation.

Provocation

> As you arrive into this book, what resonates with you in this first chapter?
> Play with that resonance through, for example, improvised movement, drawing, music, photography, roleplay and crafting.
> Shift from your experiential creative process into a short burst of free-flow writing for 3–5 minutes.
> You might want to invite a trusted colleague or friend to join you in this provocation and share your harvest.

Notes

1 Subjects, human and more-than-human, will generally be referred to by pronouns *she* or *he* (refraining from the pronoun *it*).
2 Maeve is a pseudonym. All the examples of research and practice in this book have had ethical approval from Goldsmiths, University of London, and will have been part of an official research project, with ethical approval. As such, the identity of each participant included in this book has been anonymised through a pseudonym and other potentially identifying features, such as time and place.
3 Intra-action is a term used to denote a place that is mutually implicated.
4 Assemblage is an organising concept, developed by Deleuze and Guattari (1987), bringing attention to dynamic flows between phenomena that problematise power relations.
5 Becoming, rather than being, is a liminal, in-between, ongoing process that refuses to be defined as any one particular state.
6 Chapter 6 of this book considers the process of ethical consent in relation to re-search inquiry and ecofeminist DMP practice from new materialist and posthu man perspectives.
7 The anthropocene is an era in which human activity has had an increasingly signifi-cant impact on the ecology that is now evident in the climate emergency. In line with MacCormack (2020), this is a deliberate non-capitalisation.
8 I do not wish to mention their name in this book.

References

Ahmed, S. (2010). Orientations matter. In D. Coole and S. Frost (eds.), *New Material-isms: Ontology, Agency and Politics*, pp. 234–257. London: Duke University Press.

Barad, K. (2003). Posthumanist performativity: Toward an understanding of how mat-ter comes to matter. *Signs: Journal of Women in Culture and Society*, Vol. 28, No. 3 (Gender and Science: New Issues), pp. 801–831.

Barad, K. (2012). On touching – the inhuman that therefore I am. *Differences*, Vol. 23, No. 3, pp. 206–223.

Bennett, J. (2010). *Vibrant Matter: A Political Ecology of Things*. Durham: Duke University Press.

Braidotti, R. (1997). Meta(1)morphoses. *Theory, Culture and Society*, Vol. 14, No. 2, pp. 67–80.

Deleuze, G. and Guattari, F. (1987). *A Thousand Plateaus: Capitalism and Schizophre-nia*. London: Continuum.

Frizell, C. (2023a). Bodies, landscapes, and the air that we breathe. *Kritika Kultur*, Vol. 40, pp. 66–73.

Frizell, C. (2023b). The cat, the foal and other meetings that make a difference: Post-human research that re-animates our responsiveness to knowing and becoming. In C. Frizell and M. Rova (eds.), *Creative Bodies in Therapy, Performance and Com-munity Research and Practice that Brings Us Home*, pp. 50–61. London: Routledge.

Frizell, C. and Rova, M. (eds.). (2023). *Creative Bodies in Therapy, Performance and Community Research and Practice that Brings Us Home*. London: Routledge.

Haraway, D. (2016). *Staying with the Trouble*. London: Duke University Press.

MacCormack, P. (2020). *The Ahuman Manifesto: Activism for the End of the Anthropo-cene*. London: Bloomsbury Publishing Plc.

Merleau-Ponty, M. (2004). *The World of Perception*. Oxon: Routledge.

Readfern, G. (2022). Scientists discover 'biggest plant on Earth' off Western Australian coast. *The Guardian: Environment*, Wednesday 1st June. www.theguardian.com/

environment/2022/jun/01/what-the-hell-australian-scientists-discover-biggest-plant-on-earth-off-wa-coast?CMP=Share_iOSApp_Other

Taylor, C. (2021). Knowledge matters: Five propositions concerning the reconceptualisation of knowledge in feminist new materialist, posthumanist, postqualitative approaches. In K. Murris (ed.), *Navigating the Post Qualitative New Materialist and Critical Posthumanist Terrain across Disciplines: An Introductory Guide*, pp. 22–42. London: Routledge.

Interruption 1

Have you come to see her?

I arrive in the classroom in time to greet the busy class teacher. Outside the window, a group of teaching assistants chat, their warm breath meets the cold air in clouds of condensation. They clap their gloves together and stamp their feet to keep warm as several school buses pull up in the driveway. I see Julie step down from the bus wearing black patent shoes and a checked pleated skirt that hangs beneath her pale blue, double-breasted coat. Her brown hair is brushed tightly into two long plaits that hang down her back, on either side of her rucksack. She takes the hand of a teaching assistant and continues to stare up at her as they walk towards the school entrance. Julie is the only girl amongst the eight children who hang up their coats and enter the classroom. She follows the teaching assistant to a chair in the circle and sits very still, as the other children take their time to settle. The teacher takes the register, encouraging the children to greet each other using Makaton,[1] and I am introduced as a visitor. Julie's speech is clear; however, her voice sounds flat. I am introduced and Julie looks at the floor and repeats my name twice, each time with rising intonation, emphasising the three syllables rhythmically like a nursery rhyme:

'Ca-ro-line, Ca-ro-line.'

She looks up at me with an expressionless stare. I smile, with the rhythm of my name still playing in my head. The teacher directs the children to their desks, where their tasks await them. Once they are settled, I walk over to Julie and sit on a chair at the table that she shares with two other children.

'May I sit with you, Julie.'
'Have you come to see her?' asks Julie.
'Come to see her?'
'Have you come to see Julie?'
'Oh, yes. I've come to see Julie.'
'Oh,' Julie looks at me anxiously.

On the desk in front of Julie is an A4 worksheet with a central line dividing two columns, headed *fruits* and *vegetables*. On a separate sheet of paper are colourful

DOI: 10.4324/9781003322658-3

pictures of fruits and vegetables that require cutting and sticking. The boy sitting opposite Julie looks at me and as our eyes meet, his face creases into a smile.

'How are you, Elih?' says Julie, looking out of the window.

Elih leans back into his chair and smiles, without answering.

'You seem to have some work to do,' I say, looking from Elih to Julie.
'It's Julie's work,' says Julie.

'She's got to *put* the pictures. She's got to put the *pictures*,' she repeats with a shifting emphasis.
Julie looks blankly at her work, sitting motionless with her arms holding the sides of her chair. Then she lifts her right hand and begins to tap her fingers urgently against her chin. The words *put* and *pictures* dance in my mind as isolated sounds.
'So, you've got to put the pictures . . . is that on the page?' I enquire, point-ing to the columns on the A4 paper.
Julie drops her hand down to hold the side of her chair. She looks at me expectantly and then she looks at Elih, who has already cut out an apple and carefully stuck it upside down in the *vegetables* column. The Pritt stick has left a snail trail across the table. He pats the apple several times with the palm of his hand, pauses and raises his hand to repeat the action. Julie looks back at her worksheet, still clutching the sides of her chair and says suddenly,

'How are you, Caroline? What have you been doing this week?'
'Oh,' I say, taken aback by the formality of her tone.
'Well, I was wondering the same about you.'
'Do you like Pukka pies? Julie likes Pukka pies,' she says.

The teacher's sing-song tone calls from an adjacent desk,

'Ju-lie, Ju-lie, how about some cutting and sticking . . . fruit and vegetables.'

I take that as a hint that I need to encourage Julie to focus on the activity. I pick up the sheet with the colourful pictures and a pair of scissors from the central pot on the table. I look at Julie, hoping to engage with her somehow through this activity.
Meanwhile, Elih pats the picture of the apple several times with the palm of his hand. He pauses, raises his hand and repeats the action. Looking at me, as if to check that he has my attention, he lifts his hand slowly into the air, palm downwards, and slams it down on the upside-down apple.
Bang!
Julie looks across, and for the first time she smiles.

Note

1 Makaton is a system that uses signs and gestures alongside speech to facilitate com-munication supporting people who struggle with expressive and receptive speech.

2 Creating ecofeminist perspectives through new materialist and posthuman entanglements

Maeve looks directly at me.

'I feel like I never really fulfil, er . . . fulfilled my potential.'

She looks down at her hands and lowers her voice,

'I don't even know how to tell you what it's like . . .'

Maeve's shoulders lift. Her breathing quickens. She sniffs. A tear drops onto the back of her right hand, and she quickly brushes it away.

'Sorry . . . you must think I'm so silly.'

I am touched by her emotion. I offer her the box of tissues from the table between our chairs. Maeve ignores the tissues, preferring to use the heel of her hand to wipe across one cheek and then the other. I replace the tissues on the table.

'You see, I grew up in a big family. It wasn't easy, you know. Well, it was, and it wasn't, if you know what I mean.'

Maeve takes a tissue from the box and places it on her lap. She opens it out, begins to fold it in half and then in half again. The silver-haired, smiling figure of my always-cleaning-up late grandmother comes to my mind, one of 13 children whose family migrated to London when she was a child. I imagined Maeve as a small child, surrounded by brothers and sisters in a busy, noisy household.

'When I was only just an adult,' Maeve says, 'I was *desperately* in love with this man. I would have done anything for him. And I was convinced he loved me and would leave his wife,'

DOI: 10.4324/9781003322658-4

Maeve pauses and folds the tissue in half once more.

'He said he would,' she repeats, smoothing down the folded tissue.

She looks at me. A memory flashes through my mind of sitting in class, the year Neil Armstrong set foot on the moon's surface. My friend had stood up, confidently offering a fact about space travel. The teacher asked how she knew it was true and my friend replied that it must be true because she had read it in a book. The class laughed, and my friend's humiliation squeezed into my stomach.

'I imagined the day we'd get married and how I'd be the happiest woman in the world . . .'

The words stop, as if at the edge of a cliff. Maeve looks at me frowning. Indignation rises in my chest in anticipation of a terrible hurt. I take a breath in. Maeve looks around the room. She balances the folded tissue on her lap and puts the palms of her hands on either side of her thighs, straightening her elbows to lift her weight slightly forwards towards her feet and back again, like a child on a swing.

'I would have been the happiest woman in the world,' she repeats quietly.

Maeve sits back in her chair, returns her hands to her lap and folds over a tiny corner of the tissue, smoothing it down with her index finger. I remember her neatly folded coat lying on the chair outside the studio, with the green satin lining catching the sun. She shakes her head and looks at me with a hint of irony in her smile.

'Do you know what I mean?' she asks.

Simultaneously, a concerned smile and a frown prompt the muscles in my face. I imagine broken promises and disappointments. I swallow. Maintaining eye contact, I tilt my head.

'It sounds like you felt horribly let down,' I say.
    'I did. Yes. Then, one day he cut off all contact with me. It was before we had texting and all that. He was from a different town. I didn't know where he lived, but he would phone me on the landline and send me *beautiful* letters in between our meetings. I didn't have his number because he didn't want his wife to find out. And then suddenly . . .'

Maeve pauses and folds over another corner of the tissue. She looks at me.

'He said it was over. And . . . it all . . . just stopped. It was like my life . . . just stopped.'

Maeve brings her right hand down forcefully, flattening the tissue. Her gaze is now intense and I become aware of my desire to look away.

'How terrible!' I say.

The silence is broken by the quietly ticking clock standing next to a piece of driftwood smoothed by the sea on the wooden shelf. The pain of loss grips my torso. The muscles of my face want to crumple with sadness. We continue to look at each other. She takes in a deep breath and relaxes back into her chair, taking her hand off the tissue. She then looks straight in front of her, nodding.

As if woken from a reverie, she turns her head quickly to look back at me, frowning.

'Now, why on earth was I telling you that?' she asks, in a matter-of-fact tone.

Maeve turns her head towards the sound of a crow calling outside the window. She turns back to look at the clock and then at me.

'Well,' I say.

'You were telling me that you came from a big family and, as a young adult, fell in love with a married man who then just ended the relationship, and you were left feeling hurt and distressed . . . as if life had stopped.'

I put my hand to my chest feeling the sadness.

'Ah, yes. All I remember after that is being out in the garden, barefoot in the deep snow. It must have been freezing. There was a dead blackbird lying on the ground. I picked it up and carried it to the cemetery . . .'

Maeve pauses, looking across the room at the white wall. She tilts her head to the right. My attention is caught by a rectangular patch of sunlight illuminated on the wooden floor. It disappears as the sun goes in. I imagine the lifeless black feathered body of the dead bird, one glazed eye staring up at me as it is carried to the cemetery. I get stuck in the liminal space between dreams and reality as I am alerted to Maeve's fragile psychic state some 30 years ago.

Maeve looks down at the white tissue on her lap and begins to cry. After a while, she wipes the tears from her face with the tissue, blows her nose and looks up at me.

'I felt very low for a long time,' she says.

'Mmm,' I say. 'How are you doing in your body now?'

'How am I doing in my body now?' Maeve repeats, sitting up straight and shifting further back into her chair.

'I'm not sure what you mean.'

'Well, you've told me a powerful story of your distress 30 years ago, and I wondered what that's like for you remembering that difficult experience. Now. Here. In this room. With me.'

I hear myself clumsily listing words, and I stop. I am still with the texture of the humiliation, the hurt and the psychic fragility.

'Oh, I see. Well. My heart was beating very fast as I remembered what happened, but now I feel kind of calm. Kind of relieved. Is that what you mean?'

'Well, I guess so,' I say.

Maeve laughs.

'So, I got that right then . . .. '

We both laugh spontaneously, prompted by the playfulness in Maeve's tone.

Maeve strokes the red velvet arm of the chair.

Creating and being created

We found a meeting place in that laughter: two women fumbling through an intensive and intimate intra-action. When prompted, Maeve was able to identify the real-time bodied experience of this exchange and, at the end, re-turned to the sensory comfort of the velvet cover of the chair. Maeve was telling me a potentially traumatic story and by inviting her attention into the body, I wanted to bring her into the present to prevent her becoming too overwhelmed by past trauma, bringing the process of re-membering to a manageable pace and mitigating against the risk of re-traumatisation. In these early sessions, we were developing a culture between us that included a way of practising therapy grounded in the corporeality of doing and becoming through moving bodies, rather than solely thinking and reflecting through language. This can be an unfamiliar place within Western cultures in which the experiential realm of the body becomes the subordinated other to language and discourse.

Following the shared moment of laughter that closes this vignette, I wondered out loud to Maeve how it might be to step out of the chair, away from the words and into improvisational movement, thus inviting her to move beyond representational language into the creativity of the material body. This shift from talking to moving is not always easy, and in Chapter 4, I discuss in more detail this transition and the ways in which improvisational moving bodies enliven the potential for new ways of knowing the world. In the chapter you are reading now, I will bring your attention to the ways in which new materialist and posthuman thinking can be useful in becoming immersed in material-discursive[1] landscapes in both researching and practising, towards identifying how our entangled subjectivities are embedded, embodied, nomadic and differentiating.

Creating new materialist and posthuman perspectives

When I discovered new materialism and posthumanism, I found them to be closely aligned to the work I was doing in DMP and ecopsychotherapy. The feminist philosophies of new materialist and posthuman thinkers, for example, Barad (2003, 2007, 2012, 2014), Braidotti (2013, 2019a, 2019b, 2022), and Haraway (2004, 2016), provided an effective thinking apparatus for animating my experience of the world differently, allowing 'matter its due as an active participant in the world's becoming' (Barad, 2003: 803): that is, becoming aware of the material world as alive and impactful, rather than inert and passive. These feminist thinkers draw from science and critical social theories to challenge established paradigms and discourses that underpinned Western cultural norms, troubling the kinds of knowledge that gets privileged and the ways in which power operates and becomes distributed.

New materialism,[2] as a precursor of posthumanism, evolved as a term in the late 1990s, initiated by Braidotti and DeLanda (van der Tuin & Dolphijn, 2010), providing both researching and practising with an ethico-onto-epistemological[3] rebalancing of the relationship between the materiality of intra-active bodies and language, discourse and culture. New materialism brings a focus to the significance of all matter – organic, inorganic, animate and inanimate – as performative actors in an emergent, intra-active web of relations. Furthermore, posthumanism[4] troubles ideas about what it means to be human in the first place and challenges an ideology of human exceptionalism, that is, the privileging of the desires of some humans over the needs of the wider ecological community.

Creating new materialist and posthuman intra-subjectivity

New materialist and posthuman paradigms challenge binary thinking and move towards redefining the ways in which identities are organised and sub-jectivities conceived and performed. These paradigms create innovative poten-tial for working with the affective flows of differently enabled moving bodies. Posthuman intra-subjectivity is permeable, fluid and contingent, always in an emergent process of becoming, in mutually implicated, diffracting encounters. Braidotti (1997, 2013, 2019b) developed the idea of the posthuman subject, welcoming the complexity and multiplicity of the open-ended, experiential processes of identity politics. The critical discourses of feminist identity politics help me challenge my assumptions, my choice of language and the lens that I bring to those choices as well as locating them within wider historical social, political and cultural contexts. If I can maintain an ongoing awareness of op-pressions and injustices that operate, I can begin to relate to the world and its players as an act of resistance and as part of the fabric of inclusive, rather than hostile environments. In Chapter 3, I will outline some of the theoretical foundations and praxes of intersectionality (Crenshaw, 1991) that are rooted in black feminism and political activism that called out the multiple oppres-sions of racism and sexism and challenged white feminist discourses (Bernard, 2022). These theoretical perspectives can then be effectively applied to the complex entanglements of diverse socio-political identity categories, with a view to understanding the lived experience of individuals through the lens of identity politics.

Creating assemblages

As I arrived into a relationship with Maeve, an assemblage of material bodies of all kin(ds) was emerging. New materialist and posthuman lenses enabled me, as a practitioner and researcher, to shift my perspectives on the matters that mattered, honing the craft of listening to and noticing what I might have otherwise filtered out within the emergent assemblage of relational experi-ence. This assemblage comprised the intra-personal meeting place between us, for example, Maeve's memories as they arose and as she found the words to give them a shape through language; the imaginings, memories and im-ages that were evoked in me in the presence of Maeve; the improvisational movement content; the emotional and sensory flows; the material actors in our encounters and the critical discourses that were infused into material and discursive meeting places.

In the same way that it can be hard to find the right words to contain, listen and respond to stories that any client brings to the improvisational therapy space, so, too, is it hard to find a language to represent that experience in writing. In the writing of this story, I re-enter the entanglement of this as-semblage of multiple unfolding stories. The words I select to write about the session add layers of representation, that is, how and what I choose to write, only coming part way to representing this emerging corporeal entanglement. I am reminded of the nomadic nature of improvisational moving bodies, the expression of which evades possession and refuses definition and/or measurement. Like performance, the live, improvisational encounter of the therapy session cannot be recreated and becomes itself through its transience and its disappearance. The feminist scholar and movement artist Peggy Phelan (1993) writes,

> (p)erformance's only life is in the present. Performance cannot be saved, recorded, documented, or otherwise participate in the circulation of representation of representations: once it does so, it becomes something other than performance. To the degree that performance attempts to enter the economy of reproduction, it betrays and lessens the promise of its own ontology. Performance's being . . . becomes itself through disappearance.
>
> (146)

As I read this quotation, I ponder on the idea of entering an economy of reproduction, in which the content of the session becomes research-capital, the documentation of which is in danger of betraying and lessening its ontological promise. Language takes over as the representational tool at my disposal. I begin to muse on the place of performance as a concept in therapy-as-a-process-over-time, each therapy session being part of a processual experience, that gathers momentum through different performative entanglements, which themselves are part of the performative affective economy of a material world.

My work with Maeve was itself an emergent rhizomatic assemblage in which she and I were entangled, the therapeutic process both creating and being created by multiple layers of experience. And now you, the reader, are also entangled, as you bring your own experience that diffracts into the reading of my recreation of the therapeutic encounter. You bring your own emotional responses, your associations, your critical eye, your experience and your situated material-discursive environment. There are many players entering the ongoing poetry of this assemblage and in the relational spaces between those players, boundaries can be contingent and blurred, like the patches of sunlight illuminated on the wooden floor that appear and disappear depending on how the sun, the clouds and the glass in the window frame align. Each small meeting place holds the emergent potential to know the world differently. Wyatt (2019) likens those moments of insight in the therapeutic process to the refrain in stand-up comedy, explaining how refrains

> turn and return, create and re-create, emerge and re-emerge, aslant, bearing the potential for new constellations of difference. The way coffee feels, how a door shuts in the wind, a man reaching for his water bottle, how a cat sits by a window.
>
> (94)

In my work with Maeve, there were multiple material players, such as two hu-man figures who identify as women, skin, hands, cheeks, salty tears and beat-ing hearts; an unseen crow; a shaft of sunlight on the wooden floor; a box of tissues and a single tissue that gets folded again and again; the green satin coat lining that lies across the chair outside the studio; the ticking clock keeping time next to a piece of driftwood; the white wall; the smooth red velvet of the chairs and the table that stands between them.

Then there are the players who enter through Maeve's memories: the busy family life in the rural landscape; the man who spurned her; the landline phone on which he called her and the stationary on which he wrote his love letters; the postage stamps and post box; the cold snow; the dead blackbird and the cemetery.

And then there are the players of my imagination, implicating my own stories in this entanglement: my always-cleaning-up late grandmother and her many siblings; their family story of migration from Ireland to London; my schoolgirl self, witnessing my friend's pronouncement of truth and the book that convinced her of that truth; Neil Armstrong's foot in contact with the moon's surface; the glazed eye of the lifeless blackbird staring up at me; Maeve's conviction that her lover would be true to his word; my school friend's conviction of the authority of published authors and the teacher's demand for a particular kind of evidence.

There are the emotional landscapes: that is, the feelings that shift through and between Maeve and me as we spend time together and the sadness, the indignation, the hurt, the grief, the humiliation and the laughter, all of which bring us together in intimate ever-shifting moments of connection.

Within that relational landscape, I keep an eye on the less conscious dy-namics that might be telling a story through the transferences, such as how, less consciously, for instance, Maeve might fear investing in a close and loving attachment with me arising from her experience of being spurned and once again, her life just stopping and Maeve's fear of my judgement of her state-ment *you must think I'm so silly.*

Furthermore, there are the sensory landscapes: the tactile feel of the red vel-vet and the folding and rustling of the tissue; the crow's cry, the ticking clock and the undulating rhythms and tones of the words; the gasp of the inbreath, the rush of the outbreath and a rasping sniff and blowing of the nose; and then the silence that is either waiting to appear or resisting being filled.

Then there is the landscape of critical discourses that bring issues to the foreground, such as feminism, patriarchy, anthropocentrism, religion, race, ethnicity, migration, mental health and the lens of intersectionality. These is-sues are entangled and infused both as creators and as the created within the corporeal experiences of this encounter.

In addition, there are questions of how knowledge comes to matter and what kinds of knowledge are privileged over others. My attention to the de-tails of the encounter depended on what I chose to privilege: the things that

I brought to the foreground, the things that I glossed over, the things I chose to omit and the things that hovered outside of my orbit of awareness.

And now you, the reader, bring your own unique perspective that you will be breathing into this assemblage.

The complexity of these entangled narratives invites thinking, linking and experiencing differently, that is, to foster ways of remaining spontaneous and indeterminate as we move through the tensions between creative moving bodies of all kinds, resisting notions that essentialist truths await discovery and, instead, preferring to become immersed in the eco-ethical ecology of an emergent world. Haraway (2016) alerts us to the importance of the kinds of thinking that we use and the significance of the ontologies and epistemologies that underpin our thinking. She says, '(i)t matters what stories make worlds and what worlds make stories' (12). Within those stories that we create to explain our worlds, ideas about kinship can shift our perceptive landscapes.

Creating kinship

The principles of new materialism and posthumanism can support different ways of animating subjectivity, locating the corporeality of moving bodies at their heart, in alignment with ecofeminist researching and practising that embrace social, political and ecological justice. New materialist and posthuman ontologies and epistemologies prompt a process of defamiliarisation with dominant, anthropocentric values, along with a commitment to engage with complex and often contradictory entanglements. It is a stance that urges us to move away from the exceptionalism of Eurocentric ideas about what it means to be human (and its inherent hierarchies) and to move into a more expansive identification with all matter as part of a diverse, intra-dependent ecology. Haraway (2016) suggests that kinship, as a practice, needs to move beyond ideas about ancestral or genealogical connections towards an empathic identification as live matter with an ecology of other live matter. She states,

> If there is to be multispecies ecojustice, which can also embrace diverse human people, it is high time that feminists exercise leadership in imagination, theory, and action to unravel the ties of both genealogy and kin, and kin and species.
>
> (102)

The idea of kinship and its potential to be differently imagined and differently performed optimises the possibilities of fostering climates of equality and justice.

As I sat with Maeve, the immediate material experience of the many kinds of bodies in the room was entangled with the discursive implications of the stories into which we arrived and that became created between us. This immersion in the world, as just one material body amongst many diverse bodies, brings us into an intra-active experience of *being* the world and the world *being* us. Manning (2012) uses the term *worlding* to describe this immersion, illustrating the concept with an invitation to imagine being in the garden with muddy knees, with hands digging the earth in preparation for spring planting. She challenges us with this provocation

> (i)nstead of seeing the earth as a quality apart from the knee attached to a preexisting human form, see the knee-hand-earth as a worlding, a force of form, an operative ecology.
>
> (31)

We are, at any moment, teetering on the edge of immanent and unfamiliar emergences that find kinship in diversity within an operant ecology. This kind of kinship is an experiential, material, empathic and intellectual edge of our creativity that infuses each moment with the potential of knowing the world differently, calling out,

> in the pause that precedes each breath before a moment comes into being and the world is made again.
>
> (Barad, 2007: 185)

As a practitioner, I remain alert to how this kinship might manifest. In a previous publication (Frizell, 2020), I present the story of Eric, a learning-disabled boy, with whom I worked as a DMP. I recount one session when a woodlouse entered the therapeutic space, triggering Eric's projection of his feelings of vulnerability and helplessness onto the insect, who became a target for his rage. This rage then shifted to curiosity in an inexplicable, intra-active moment of insight when Eric began to identify with the defenceless woodlouse, who he subsequently invited into his playhouse. A process of deterritorialisation[5] (Deleuze & Guattari, 1987) was in operation as Eric disidentified with an anthropocentric dominion and became open to the talismanic power of the woodlouse in a 'posthuman interconnectedness' (Braidotti, 1997: 71). Eric connected to an expanded sense of himself as a human subject, extending an empathic kinship to a member of the insect world. Braidotti (ibid) refers to the 'destabilizing posthuman speed' (74) of the impressively rapid transformative and adaptive capacities of insects that, she says, serve as an inspiration to the potentiality of becoming. The story of Eric's meeting with the woodlouse illustrates how worlds can become animated differently in the embracing of all matter 'as an active participant in the world's becoming' (Barad, 2003: 803). Such encounters (re)position human subjects as embedded, embodied and nomadic, living in (and among and as) *spacetimematter*.[6] The affective, relational flows of matter-in-the-becoming are places of intra-action, that is, of being created by the experiences that we are simultaneously creating.

I am aware that the language used to articulate processes of relational, material bodies through new materialist and posthuman lenses can become very dense and, at times, impenetrable. The terminology itself can, in fact, present difficulties, creating tensions within webs of representational language. In order to support some of the terminologies used in this book, I have added a number of explanatory notes and I have created a 'List of terms' in the prelims. In fact, the writing of the 'List of terms' was also a useful process that I would recommend. The 'List of terms' is not so much a definition of words but rather a reference point to consider the relevance of concepts as dynamic processes in researching and practising.

Creating terminology

New materialism and posthumanism cannot be neatly explained through a list of static concepts and terminologies. Authors, researchers and practitioners have played with creating neologisms[7] in their struggle with using representational language to communicate the complexity of the terminologies. For example, Ringrose et al. (2019) created the neologism PhEmaterialism to reflect the multiplicities of bringing together ideas from new materialism, posthumanism and ecofeminism within educational research – the capital *E* emphasising education. Allegranti (2021) plays further with this idea, creating the word PheMaterialism (the capital M emphasising materiality) to traverse multiple material affective, relational landscapes. Taylor (2021) concertinas feminist new materialist, posthumanist and postqualitative approaches into an acronym FNMPHPQ. The point of these examples is that the concepts represent multiple and complex ideas, and the component parts do not make sense in isolation, and neither are they static or fixed. These examples of neologisms invite terminologies that are fluid and dynamic, whilst also remaining rigorous in discourses that are grounded in ethical, ontological and epistemological principles that support anti-oppressive thinking. In the same way that ecofeminism is not a definitive, agreed term by a homogenous group called *ecofeminists*, new materialism and posthumanism are dynamic terms, creating discourses that provoke debate, rather than creating a homogenous group of thinkers. The fluidity in the semantics of these ideas is processual, that is, shapeshifting and always in the process of becoming something new. In that sense, they can also be frustratingly elusive, particularly when we seek definitive meanings. Ideas that are always in the making resist becoming hegemonic linguistic dogma and, instead, are part of democratic discourses that support different ways of thinking about and performing social identities. I wonder how you might play with the terminologies in this book, creating your own neologisms that stimulate different perspectives and vertices from which to experience the world.

The irony is that the complexity of the terminology that seeks to become rooted in the materiality of the world can then make for critiques and discourses that can become exclusive, inaccessible and disembodied. I can find that in the struggle to find a language that reflects the complexity of a dynamic experience, I find myself moving away from the materiality of my sensing, feeling, intuiting and bodily experience of the world into the conceptualising activity of my intellect.

Thank goodness for the improvising dance that can ground these abstractions of the intellect in my material presence in the world. As I dance, I participate in the world within an ever-changing 'sensory-kinetic palette of possibilities' (LaMothe, 2015: 57) – the significance is in the experience. I can find that as I shift my focus into language and discourse, it is easy for the materiality of the experience to become lost in representative language. Holding on to both (the material and the discursive), simultaneously, is no mean feat.

Creating (in)conclusive thoughts

The principles of ecofeminism, grounded in new materialism and posthumanism, do not take subjectivities for granted, and as Maeve and I worked together, subjectivity was a material-discursive emergent process, rather than a pre-existing entity that awaited discovery. Braidotti (2022) describes this kind of transversal thinking as creating chains of solidarity, remaining open and available to differently lived realities that become illuminated in relational and diffractive meeting places. The posthuman subject is embedded, embodied, nomadic and differentiating, entangled in the matter(ing) of material-discursive phenomena. That chain of solidarity is immersed in the diversity of post(not just)human bodies. This notion of posthuman subjectivity invites a defamiliarisation with anthropocentrism and a disidentification with dominant patriarchal cultural values.

Ecofeminism through new materialist and posthumanist lenses challenges human exceptionalism inherent in anthropocentrism that privileges the subjectivity of being a particular kind of human (the 'I,' the 'we' and the 'who' that identify with particular attributes) over the objectivity of being not human (the 'it,' the 'them' and the 'that,' being deficient of those attributes). Critical discourses offer me different lenses with which I can begin to make connections between the personal and the political and link the unique story of, for example, one woman to the wider ideologies, myths and discourses of our time.

Within the evolution of socio-political structures in the Western world, the subjectivity of some humans has been privileged over others within binary hierarchical structures that create dominant and subordinate categories. Black Lives Matter (BLM), the #MeToo movement, disability activism and LGBTQ+ activism are examples of movements that highlight and expose historical structural oppressions and inequalities. These movements hold potential for redefining subjectivity as we shift from binaries into multiplicities towards what Braidotti (2019b) describes as 'transversal subjectivity' (161).

Maeve alluded to her perception of her own insignificance, for example, when she claimed that I would think she was *just silly*. At the beginning of our process together, she struggled to find her agency as an affective actor in a relational affect economy, particularly regarding gender and class. Maeve doubted that her life was of importance. However, the act of stepping into therapy suggested that Maeve's less conscious activist spirit suspected that things *could* be different and this might be seen as a less conscious, inner drive to challenge the oppressions that she had internalised. This therapeutic entanglement was an opportunity for Maeve to animate her perception and her experience of her place in the world differently.

And at the end of this chapter, I leave you with a provocation to reflect on this assemblage of ideas.

Provocation

> How do you, the reader, move through ideas about being just one (small) part of an active, living world that is always going on?
>
> I invite you to spend some time engaging in a creative process in response to this question and then finish with a spontaneous burst of free-flow writing.
>
> If you have a peer, friend or colleague to hand, spend some time sharing your thoughts together. What are the similarities and differences in your responses?

Notes

1 The term *material-discursive* as a hyphenated neologism was coined by the feminist physicist and philosopher Barad (2007), referring to the mutually constituted nature of materiality (i.e., the physical presence of phenomena) and discourse (the representative thinking linked to phenomena).
2 For examples of authors addressing new materialism, see Barad (2003, 2007, 2012, 2014), Barrett (2013), Coole & Frost (2010), Davies (2010, 2014, 2017, 2021), Fox & Alldred (2015, 2017) and Ringrose et al. (2019).
3 Barad (2007) creates the neologism *ethico-onto-epistemology* by conflating the terms ethics (i.e., the way justice is thought about and applied), ontology (the nature of existing in the world) and epistemology (the parameters within which knowledge emerges), suggesting that they cannot be separated as each is dependent on the others.
4 For examples of authors addressing posthumanism, see Braidotti (2013, 2019, 2022), Murris (2021a, 2021b) and Taylor (2021).
5 Territorialisation and deterritorialisation are terms conceived by Deleuze and Guattari (1987) as processes that create oppositional forces of stability in systems that are then destabilised by lines of flight that deviate from a predictable trajectory. This process of disruption shifts the normativity inherent in belief systems and assumptions to create new ways of thinking about and organising practices, for example, those underpinning binary oppositional pairs of dominating and subordinating hierarchies.
6 *Spacetimematter* is a neologism created by Barad (2007) to describe the entangled relationship between space, time and matter. Each is non-static and diffracts across and enfolds into the other in a continuously moving intra-active engagement.
7 A neologism is a newly created word, phrase and/or acronym, often created from an existing word or words that create(s) a line of flight into new concepts and meanings, usually bringing together multiple ideas.

References

Allegranti, B. (2021). Dancing activism. In H. Wengrower and S. Chaiklin (eds.), *Dance and Creativity within Dance Movement Therapy: International Perspectives*, pp. 157–177. New York/Oxon: Routledge.

Barad, K. (2003). Posthumanist performativity: Toward an understanding of how matter comes to matter. *Signs: Journal of Women in Culture and Society*, Vol. 28, No. 3 (Gender and Science: New Issues), pp. 801–831.

Barad, K. (2007). *Meeting the Universe Halfway: Quantum Physics and the Entanglement of Matter and Meaning*. London: Duke University Press.

Barad, K. (2012). On touching – the inhuman that therefore I am. *Differences*, Vol. 23, No. 3, pp. 206–223.

Barad, K. (2014). Diffracting diffraction: Cutting together-apart. *Parallax*, Vol. 20, No. 3, pp. 168–187.

Barrett, E. (2013). Materiality, affect, and the aesthetic image. In E. Barrett and B. Bolt (eds.), *Carnal Knowledge: Towards a 'New Materialism' through the Arts*, pp. 63–72. London: I.B. Tauris.

Bernard, C. (2022). *Intersectionality for Social Workers: A Practical Introduction to Theory and Practice*. Oxon: Routledge.

Braidotti, R. (1997). Meta(1)morphoses. *Theory, Culture and Society*, Vol. 14, No. 2, pp. 67–80.

Braidotti, R. (2019a). A theoretical framework for the critical posthumanities. *Theory, Culture and Society*, Vol. 36, No. 6, pp. 31–61.

Braidotti, R. (2019b). *Posthuman Knowledge*. Cambridge: Polity Press.

Braidotti, R. (2013). *The Posthuman*. Cambridge: Polity.

Braidotti, R. (2022). *Posthuman Feminism*. Cambridge: Polity Press.

Coole, D. and Frost, S. (eds.). (2010). *New Materialisms: Ontology, Agency and Politics*. London: Duke University Press.

Crenshaw, K. (1991). Mapping the margins: Intersectionality, identity politics, and violence against women of color. *Stanford Law Review*, Vol. 43, No. 6, pp. 1241–1299.

Davies, B. (2010). The implications for qualitative research methodology of the struggle between the individualised subject of phenomenology and the emergent multiplicities of the poststructuralist subject: The problem of agency. *Reconceptualizing Educational Research Methodology*, Vol. 1, No. 1, p. 54.

Davies, B. (2014). Reading anger in early childhood intra-actions: A diffractive analysis. *Qualitative Inquiry*, Vol. 20, No. 6, pp. 734–741.

Davies, B. (2017). Animating ancestors: From representation to diffraction. *Qualitative Inquiry*, Vol. 23, No. 4, pp. 267–275.

Davies, B. (2021). *Entanglement in the World's Becoming and the Doing of New Materialist Inquiry*. New York: Routledge.

Deleuze, G. and Guattari, F. (1987). *A Thousand Plateaus: Capitalism and Schizophrenia*. London: Continuum.

Fox, N. and Alldred, P. (2015). New materialist social inquiry: Designs, methods and the research-assemblage. *International Journal of Social Research Methodology*, Vol. 18, No. 4, pp. 399–414.

Fox, N. and Alldred, P. (2017). *Sociology and the New Materialism*. London: Sage.

Frizell, C. (2020). Reclaiming our innate vitality: Bringing embodied narratives to life through dance movement psychotherapy. In A. Williamson and B. Sellers-Young (eds.), *Spiritual Herstories: Call of the Soul in Dance Research*, pp. 207–220. Bristol: Intellect.

Haraway, D. (2004). Modest_Witness@Second_Millennium. In D. Haraway (ed.), *The Haraway Reader*, pp. 223–250. New York: Routledge.

Haraway, D. (2016). *Staying with the Trouble*. London: Duke University Press.

LaMothe, K. (2015). *Why We Dance: A Philosophy of Bodily Becoming*. New York: Columbia University Press.

Manning, E. (2012). *Always More Than One: Individuation's Dance*. Durham: Duke University Press.

Murris, K. (ed.). (2021a). Making kin: Postqualitative, new materialist and posthumanist research. In K. Murris (ed.), *Navigating the Postqualitative New Materialist and Critical Posthumanist Terrain across Disciplines: An Introductory Guide*, pp. 1–21. Oxon: Routledge.

Murris, K. (2021b). The 'missing peoples' of critical posthumanism and new materialism. In K. Murris (ed.), *Navigating the Postqualitative New Materialist and Critical Posthumanist Terrain across Disciplines: An Introductory Guide*, pp. 62–84. Oxon: Routledge, 2021.

Phelan, P. (1993). *Unmarked*. London: Routledge

Ringrose, J., Warfield, K. and Zarabadi, S. (eds.). (2019). *Feminist Posthumanisms, New Materialisms and Education*. London: Routledge.

Taylor, C. (2021). Knowledge matters: Five propositions concerning the reconceptualisation of knowledge in feminist new materialist, posthumanist, postqualitative approaches. In K. Murris (ed.), *Navigating the Postqualitative New Materialist and Critical Posthumanist Terrain across Disciplines: An Introductory Guide*, pp. 22–42. London: Routledge.

van der Tuin, I. and Dolphijn, R. (2010). The transversality of new materialism, *Women: A Cultural Review*, Vol. 21, No. 2, pp. 153–171.

Wyatt, J. (2019). *Therapy, Stand-Up, and the Gesture of Writing*. London: Routledge.

Interruption 2

The guises of blessings

I sat in a carriage of a Piccadilly line tube train on my way to Great Ormond Street Hospital, holding my baby swaddled to my chest. The infant was on regular doses of medication, fed by a tube, and her heart was failing. Shortly after birth, there had been a catastrophic diagnosis. A heart operation could not be carried out before she was a sufficient weight, and without an operation, she would die, we were told. Statistically, the success rate of the operation was poor. *It was probably for the best*, they had said, *a blessing in disguise, given the learning disability.* The baby was reaching 3 months, and the appointment was to discuss the pending operation.

I held her close and became aware of an attentive figure standing by me in the crowded train. Looking up, I met with the eyes of a stranger. His skin was smooth. His cropped, jet-black hair stood on end, framing a compassionate gaze. I was on the verge of averting my eyes, and he said,

'Your baby is very ill.'
'Yes,' I said, defensively, taken aback by his comment.

Feeling conspicuous, I glanced around the carriage. In my mind's eye, I returned (to) the moment that the paediatrician had broken the news that the baby had Down's syndrome by pointing out the characteristic features, as if examining a medical specimen. The stranger's silent attention compelled me to look back up. He was waiting with a gentle smile.

'I can heal your baby. She has a bad heart. I can heal it.'

Without explanation, he clasped his hands above me-with-the-baby-swaddled-to-my-chest and spoke in a soft, singing voice. I looked from the stranger to my baby and back again, suspended in a spacetimematter confusion. I glanced around the carriage, feeling exposed and humiliated, but thankfully found that this performance remained an insignificance to other passengers. Nevertheless, I needed it to stop.

'I really think . . .' I began, looking back towards the stranger, but he was not there.

DOI: 10.4324/9781003322658-5

The train door was open, and passengers jostled for position. There was standing room only.

***

The tiny baby lay on the treatment bed, and the consultant listened through his stethoscope, tilting his head. His body was motionless. He turned to scrutinise his scans, as if desperately searching for something he had lost. I braced myself, anticipating more difficult news. This was the consultant whose eyes had filled with tears when he first diagnosed the heart problem. He was a man full of love.

'This . . . seems . . . remarkable . . .' he was stumbling over his words.
'The heart seems to have rectified itself . . . let me check again . . .'

In my mind's eye, I flung open the doors of the tube train, shouting for the stranger to return and explain his mischief.

Thirty-six years later, I receive a text from the manager of the community home. It says, simply,

'She is a breath of fresh air.'

Guises of blessings held contradiction and paradox. A line of flight carried me into experiencing new worlds differently.

3 Equality, diversity and inclusion

Disability (for example) as a marker of difference

Sitting at an oblique angle to each other, my attention wanders as Maeve speaks. It is hard to follow the storyline. My mind scrambles to find connections, to ascertain meaning and to follow a plot. Anxiety rises in my torso. I replay the moment last week when she had become upset by my witnessing her movement. *Please don't look at me*, she had said, tears rolling down her cheeks. *The shame is overwhelming*, she had said – shame about her body, shame about who she is and shame of not being enough. The shame of who she imagines she becomes in my eyes. Then today, she says, it was hard to turn up. I find myself identifying with the projection of the inattentive listener, perhaps the unavailable mother.

Maeve is still speaking. I take my weight onto my right elbow, pushing into the arm of the chair, and as I shift position, I begin to connect to anxiety in my torso. I give it some attention, turning to face it, rather than trying to shift away from it, and the anxiety races through my ribs and rises into my jaw. As it lessens, I realise that underneath is the shame of not knowing how to connect or respond to Maeve's monologue. The shame creeps up uncomfortably across my skin, pricking either side of my neck. My jaw feels tense. I swallow, and at that moment, as I allow the uncomfortable feelings some space inside me, I begin to connect emotionally to the story that Maeve is telling me. She continues,

> '. . . so I took some flowers to his house to apologise. When he saw it was me, he closed the door in my face. I felt so ashamed. I went home and tried to phone him . . . but he didn't answer, and I never saw him again. I just don't know how I could get it so wrong.'

Maeve leans forwards and clasps her hands together. She puts her elbows on her knees and fixes her gaze in mine, as if intuiting that she now has

DOI: 10.4324/9781003322658-6

my full attention. I sit back in my seat and hold her gaze, feeling moved by the image of this brutal rejection.

'. . . how could I get it so wrong?' she asks.
'It seems like there was a painful misunderstanding between you.'

I linger on the words *painful misunderstanding*. I am now immersed in Maeve's experience.

Differing vertices

At first, I noticed that it was hard to engage with Maeve in this session. Her initial complex monologue was perhaps a defence against feeling the shame of not being enough. I, too, seemed to be defending against connecting to Maeve's emotional experience, and I perhaps got caught up less consciously in identifying with a powerful projection. Either way, a chasm was created that was hard to bridge. When I gave my anxiety some attention, as it manifested in my physical, emotional and sensory experience, I noticed how it was masking more difficult feelings. Somewhat reluctantly, I managed to locate the uncomfortable countertransferential[1] shame, in some of its many different shades, that was constellating in the emotional field. The shame and vulnerability resonated on some level with my own experience, and it took me some time to get hold of this in the communication.

That sense of not being enough is just one symptom of a complex system of values of worth, within neoliberal identity politics of advanced capitalism that privileges particular abilities and values, such as economic productivity, academic acuity, independence and the capacity for material consumption over and above, for example, kindness, care and compassion. In a competitive market, ability is a central marker of success, for example, in educational institutions, in working environments and in leisure pursuits. Measures of worth have historically privileged able-bodied, male, affluent, well-educated, heteronormative, white European embodiments of the human and are the residue of our colonial past. Maeve was carrying some powerful internalised projections about who she was as a working-class, menopausal-woman-getting-older, single parent, who was also a migrant. These projections had become part of her performativity in relation to the complexity of internalised social identities.

The activist in me listened through the lens of the body politic that connects the narratives that are unique to the individual with wider structural, socio-political inequalities and oppressions that are systemic. We can return to our own stories again and again from different vertices, each time bringing to light new perspectives and new understandings. Intersectional theoretical perspectives can then illuminate how structural inequalities and discrimination manifest in the lived experience of individuals at the intersections of multiple social identities, such as gender, race, class, disability, age, sexual orientation, mental health and many more. The intersections of these social categories are transversal bodied meeting places that become potent markers of difference. The theory of intersectionality can be a useful tool for critical thinking within practice and research.

Differences and the complexities of intersectionality

Crenshaw (1991) coined the term intersectionality, challenging and articulating the ways in which feminist identity politics failed to acknowledge the complexity of lived differences, particularly regarding race. Focusing solely on the issues of one singular social category as a homogenous group, such as women, fails to recognise the additional impact of, for example, race on that experience. Crenshaw (ibid) writes:

> Feminist efforts to politicize experiences of women and antiracist efforts to politicize experiences of people of color have frequently proceeded as though the issues and experiences they each detail occur in mutually exclusive terrains. Although racism and sexism readily intersect in the lives of real people, they seldom do in feminist and antiracist practices. And so, when the practices expound identity as woman or person of color as an either/or proposition, they relegate the identity of women of color to a location that resists telling.
>
> (1242)

This was a call to move away from binary thinking (i.e., either/or) towards joined-up thinking that recognises the complex power imbalances experienced by people marginalised by both gender and race. Bernard (2022) describes how intersectionality was rooted in the experience of black feminists as a response to a (predominantly white) feminist movement that privileged gender as a homogenous social category, without consideration of additional oppressions that were experienced through race. Bernard (ibid) summaries how intersectionality as a theoretical tool supported an understanding of the racialising of gendered experiences of black women in relation to gender-based violence. The three dimensions of this comprised, firstly, structural intersectionality, such as socio-economic factors and institutional discrimination; secondly, political intersectionality, such as how multiply oppressed individuals found themselves at the margins of organised activism; and thirdly, representational intersectionality that challenged discourses stigmatising black women. Intersectionality, as a theoretical and methodological tool, whilst rooted in critical race theory, can also be applied more widely in relation to multiply marginalised social identities, such as those defined by the Equality Act of 2010,[2] that is, age, disability, gender reassignment, marriage and civil partnership, race, religion and belief, sex and sexual orientation and, in addition, but not included in this legislation, class, mental health status, migrant status, care-experienced young people, those in the criminal justice system, Gypsy, Roma and Traveller (GRT) communities and other social identities that you, the reader, might identify. All these social identities can be a target for implicit and explicit discriminations.

Intersectionality has supported my thinking in relation to structural, political and representational injustices and inequalities as I work as a researcher, practitioner, educator and writer. I can, however, sometimes struggle to locate my voice within a discourse that is rooted in black feminism, and I remain aware of what I represent in terms of skin colour, socio-economic status, (dis)ability, sexual orientation and age. I find that I get caught in a tension between my commitment to anti-oppressive language and practice as a practitioner, researcher and educator and an awareness that my social identity, in terms of how my whiteness, my middle-classness, my able-bodied-ness and my heterosexuality, for example, represents oppressive privileges of social identity. This is a complex arena. I find that as I grow older, alongside that privilege that I inhabit, I am increasingly aware of the subtle dimensions of how ageism and gender discrimination intersect within that lived experience. In addition, as the parent of a learning-disabled adult, a carer for a sibling and previously a carer for parents with deteriorating health as they reached the end of their lives, I have been immersed in the politics of disability, yet can also find myself on the margins of disability activism due to my immediate social identity of being able-bodied.

As an ecofeminist, and also as an advocate for disability rights, I can find myself caught within intersectional tensions in terms of social justice. For example, a woman's choice in relation to reproductive rights can sit at odds with the rights and equal opportunities of disabled people, for example, with reference to legislation for the termination of pregnancies. This tension, along with the raw lived experience of potential dilemmas, is explored in the Channel 4 documentary entitled 'Disability and Abortion: The Hardest Choice.'[3] It is presented by actors Ruth Madeley, who has spina bifida, and Ruben Reuter, who has Down's syndrome. The presenters engage with the debates and dilemmas about prenatal screening, including the possibility of aborting a foetus after 24 weeks, which is legally possible if a significant disability is detected (such as those experienced by the presenters of the programme). These are impactful markers of difference, and the intersections open up spaces to consider the complexities of inequalities and oppressions that are sometimes hard to reconcile.

Intersectionality is a sticky web of meeting places. I wonder what your stories are, and what it is like for you to locate your voice within discourses of intersectionality.

Differences as markers

As I spent time with Maeve, I was aware of the specificity of her experience in terms of, for example, gender, class, age and migrant status and the convergence of the different intersections that had contributed to her sense of her own worth and her self-deprecation. In that brief moment, described at the beginning of this chapter, the shame that ricocheted between us held wider stories of structural oppressions. Maeve's family of origin was dominated by volatile male energies, shaping her perception and experience of significant relationships. Her sense of entitlement and her employment opportunities have been shaped and impacted by class, gender, age, migrant and marital status. In addition, Maeve was experiencing some debilitating effects of menopause and the accompanying gender-specific ageism of becoming an older woman. Mental health struggles arise within matrices that comprise the specificity of an individual's experience and the powerful interplay of identity politics and systemic socio-political injustices, inequalities and oppressions.

Being just human enough, or not, has been used to justify and normalise inequalities and oppressions. For example, during the COVID-19 pandemic, learning-disabled people died disproportionally due to inequalities in health and social care. In wider contexts, the hierarchical characteristics of white colonialism have been used to justify unspeakable racialist, sexist, homophobic and ableist violence towards groups of peoples, as well as to uphold environmental injustices. Social categories become markers of difference within ideologies through which powerful conscious and less conscious discrimination becomes enacted. For example, the eugenics society, founded by Frances Galton in 1907, developed ideas about *improving* the human race, justifying sterilisation and segregating those considered *feeble-minded*. Learning disability is indeed a powerful marker of difference and carries with it an historical legacy of oppression.

I remember visiting the Museum of Terrors in Berlin, a place of remembrance on the site of the Nazi Party central command. Amidst the many horrendous stories of the holocaust of World War II, I stood in front of a poster portraying a confused-looking disabled man sitting on a chair, legs tucked awkwardly beneath him, left shoulder raised and left arm twisted onto his lap. A white-coated doctor stood behind him, resting his hands paternally on both shoulders of the seated man. The doctor's gentle, paternal smile directed at the camera was chilling. The poster was propaganda that identified the disabled man as the passive *other*, unproductive and financially burdensome within an ableist ideology that considers disability as nothing more than a drain on society. A wave of grief surged through me as I stood, transfixed, by this compelling image, hot tears pricking the backs of my eyes. I was caught between a compulsion to confront this terrible image and the urge to flee and to convince myself with a placation that things are different these days. The image of the man in that poster embodies the stigma, suffering and impairment that are projected onto disability: what Mitchel and Snyder (2015) refer to as 'the radical vulnerability of embodiment' (7). This nationalist image of ableism upholds a way of inhabiting the body politic that creates markers of differences within frames of normativity.

Differently abled

Learning disability as a marker of difference has informed a significant amount of my practising and researching. I am (admittedly) driven by the lived experience of disability through the birth of my own daughter with Down's syndrome over three and a half decades ago, which led me through an experiential, rhizomatic labyrinth towards critical disability studies as a scholarship that has underpinned my writing, researching and practising. On the one hand, I am cautious that my own lived experience might manifest in an over-identification that clouds my capacity to see, hear, sense and think about disability. On the other hand, the lived experience as knowledge experience provides a motivation and drive to address disability justice and provides me with finely (at)tuned antennae to everyday issues of discrimination.

The process of othering of the disabled body in an ableist culture is pervasive. The meeting on the tube train in *Interruption 2: The guises of blessings* (pages 39–40) that precedes this chapter was a moment of diffraction[4] that reset the 'spacetimemattering' (Barad, 2007: 169) of my worlding compass, highlighting the intra-active, inseparable relationship between space, time and matter and in which bodies are dynamic performers. The experience of parenting a learning-disabled daughter has kept me closely in touch with disability injustices and discrimination, and to this day, I keep my activist voice on a gentle simmer. For example, in my previous writing (Frizell, 2023a), I illustrate the way in which accessing disability support and benefits, itself, is a disempowering and disenfranchising experience. In the writing, I craft a material-discursive critique of the experience of waiting on the end of a disability helpline, as a crisis in care results in my daughter's social care breaking down.

Ryan (2019) unveils some shocking truths about the oppression of disabled people in the UK, who find themselves the subject of a notion that

> still widely associates disability with tragedy and perpetuates an individual analysis for something that is fundamentally structural.
>
> (8)

Slorach (2016) argues that disability is a form of social oppression, which has been shaped by capitalism as

> professions and industries classified, regulated and graded individual human capacities according to their relationship with production. The new world . . . justified and promoted discrimination against social groups identified as different or as a threat to new social norms.
>
> (92)

Neoliberal values in an advanced capitalist system have a narrow focus on productivity and economic growth as priorities, and within those values, disability as a lived experience can become a place in which injustices and oppressions become enacted.

Difference as potential

Disability, however, is a place of possibility and potential in which the idea of ability can be reimagined to embrace intra-dependent flows of affective possibilities within the diffractive meeting places of diversely moving bodies. The multiple dimensions and body politics of our entangled moving bodies are manifestations of ideological, social, political and cultural power relations, as much as they are biological matter. I came across the disability activist and author Judith Snow at an inclusive education conference in the 1980s. Snow (1994) asserted that there are two simple gifts which belong to all of us: *presence* and *diversity*. The gift of *presence* offers a relational potential by virtue of our very existence; if we can breathe, we have a part to play. To be alive, in whatever way that might be, is to be present. The gift of *diversity* offers each unique difference as a portal to the creative potential of community. The greater the difference, the greater the potential. The powerful simplicity of these ethical principles has remained with me as a touchstone throughout my career. The combined gifts of presence and diversity are rooted in a deep reverence for all life and create opportunities for meaningful connection, as we come to find ways of caring for all others. As we meet with the differences in each other, we meet with opportunities to find new ways of being with each other. In the 1990s, Snow offered an optimistic message about the pursuit of rights, rather than charity, for differently moving bodies.

Differently moving bodies

The disabled body does not conform to ableist norms and inhabits a presence on the periphery (Mitchel & Snyder, 2015) of a normalised ideal of what bodies should be like and how bodies should move. Disabled dancer David Toole defied ableist norms in the professional dance world,[5] challenging choreographers, dancers and audiences to reimagine the possibilities of dance performance. As a young child, David had both legs amputated and went on to become a professional dancer who brought new and innovative possibilities of movement practice into dance performance. David's career was also a statement challenging the 'privileges of citizenship' (Mitchel & Snyder, 2015: 17). Differently empowered bodies trouble normative and idealised notions of how bodies should perform. Mitchel and Snyder (ibid) consider how the 'zones of bodily and affective imperfections' (ibid: 39) are targeted by the commercial media, as our bodily insufficiencies 'multiply across every surface, crevice, and cavity of the personal interior and exterior spaces of embodiment' (ibid). Normalised states of health become part of our bodily experience as we come to know ourselves in terms of what is missing, malfunctioning and deficient.

In systems within health, education, social and community services, there are notions of wholeness and coherence that create horizons of desirability. At times, Maeve was consumed with shame about perceiving herself as falling short of the desirable body. To perform being human in a way that denotes wholeness and coherence is laden with discourses of the body politic. Our relationship with (our) bodies is colonised by the commercial media, locating problems in the individual, rather than systemically. Mitchel and Snyder (2015) state,

> Neoliberal politics references all bodies as deficient and in the need of supplementations to treat the inbuilt inferiority within, a system of bodily referencing shorn of environmental causes.
>
> (39–40)

I remember pushing my learning-disabled daughter's pram into a mother and baby shop to be struck by notions of the idealised baby human all around me. Within the subtle folds of a consumer culture, as the mother of a baby diagnosed as learning-disabled I remember the uncomfortable, silent isolation that I felt. The disabled baby finds that the matter of her very particular characteristics attracts a particular gaze. Hickey-Moody (2009) notes how learning-disabled people are subject to particular social coding through medical discourses. She says that

> (m)edical discourses construct social faces of people with intellectual disability through attributing particular significances to their physical features and arguing these are signs of a specific kind of subjectivity.
>
> (13)

Medical discourses are entangled in perceptions of subjectivity in relation to disability. Actor Sarah Gordy (2020) recalls the numerous occasions when she has had to assuage the anxiety of television directors as she realised their lack of confidence in her capacity to fulfil her role as an actor, finding herself positioned in a very particular way due to having Down's syndrome. She states,

> I am a woman and an actor first. I have Down's syndrome, but that's not all I am. There is so much more to me than my disability.
>
> (55)

Shakespeare (2013) describes an historical shift to a social model of disability, which is a term coined by Oliver (1983) to shift the emphasis from a medical model of fixing individual impairments to a model that seeks to provide accessible, facilitating environments that accommodate different impairments. The shift in focus, therefore, was towards the systemic and structural barriers to participation. Shakespeare identifies problems at political and conceptual levels in the binary thinking of medical models versus social models, as individuals' subjective experiences are complex both medically *and* socially. Medical intervention certainly has the potential to improve quality of life, and individual experiences of difference cannot be magically alleviated by a formulaic manipulation of the environment. New materialist and posthuman ontologies and epistemologies can throw light on issues of disability as complex material-discursive phenomena through which the multiplicity of embodied experience is an interplay among individual subjectivity, medical perspectives *and* the environment *and* the historical discourses that have evolved.

This othering of groups of peoples is ontologically and epistemologically embedded within subtle cultural folds and it can be hard to find an emancipatory language with which to speak about learning disability in the struggle against pervasive normative forces that create, and are created by, the language available to us. This language often projects notions of vulnerability onto disabled people. Language around disability reflects the reality that some bodies have come to matter less within an ableist culture that subordinates disability as *other*. LIddiard et al. (2019) argue for a dishuman perspective for thinking about disability that challenges the humanism that is

> associated with the birth of a citizenry deemed able to speak and write with eloquence and clarity.
>
> (1475)

The posthumanities question what it is we mean by the very term *human* and a dishuman perspective resists the homogenisation of subjectivities.

Differently languaged

The term disability is not a neutral term and derogatory language in relation to learning disability can be found in the common vernacular, as illustrated by micro-aggressive insults that reference cognitive, physical, sensory or mental health impairments. In 2022, the official annual digital statistics published by the NHS[6] used the term 'mental retardation' to refer to learning disability, which is generally considered offensive (Thomas, 2022). Furthermore, problematic stereotypes reside in language that projects tragedy and vulnerability onto disability, as well as that which idealises the achievements of disabled people as courageous and/or inspirational. Derogatory and stereotypical language constitutes a form of othering that sets disabled people apart (Andrews et al., 2019). Ziegler (2020) notes how

> stigmatizing language used to label and describe individuals with disabilities has historically emphasized inferiority and otherness.
>
> (1186)

The language we use to speak about disability is charged with this legacy of diagnosis, medicalisation and discrimination. The ability/disability binary lends itself to othering, despite the fact that most people do not fit into one category or the other (Slorach, 2016). We all have dependency needs and it is important to find a language that reflects this. Disability is everyone's concern, yet disabled people carry the weight of this concern.

I shifted from using the term *people with learning disabilities* (i.e., people first) to *learning-disabled people* (i.e., people disabled by the environment) in order to align to the social model of disability that locates the disabling factors in the context, rather than the individual. Debates about terminologies in relation to learning disability might serve as displaced distress and discomfort about the subject that is less easy to think about, feel or articulate (Sinason, 2010). I sense a discomfort in my body in relation to the power and the inadequacy of language, particularly in relation to a group of people, many of whom find the privileging of language as a dominant mode of communication to be a barrier to full participation.

Differently vulnerable moving bodies

In a dream,

> *I descend a staircase in a wheelchair. Another wheelchair user is ahead of me. I struggle with the precarious decent and began to fall, seemingly out of control, and I grab the rail next to the staircase. The wheelchair falls from beneath me, clattering downstairs. I cling to the rail, disabled by the loss of the wheelchair.*

Reflecting on this dream, I wondered what it meant for myself, currently identifying as able-bodied, to dream of being disabled. The dream seemed to be a powerful message about the disabling impact of removing essential support; that is, my being a wheelchair user and having that wheelchair taken away is a powerful metaphor for my vulnerability hovering beneath the essential systems of support that sustain my participation. We are all vulnerable when we are denied essential support that enables us to participate fully in the world. Disability confronts us with the vulnerability of embodiment (Mitchel & Snyder, 2015), which is an issue that belongs to us all.

In the UK, the financial crash of 2008 triggered welfare reforms that heralded an era of austerity. Community care grants and crisis loans were abolished. Services for disabled people were either reduced or stopped (Ryan, 2019). Woven into this narrative was the notion of disability benefit fraud and Ryan articulates how the message that seeped subtly into the sociopolitical arena was that the recession had been caused by a welfare bill that had been inflated by benefit scroungers pretending to be disabled, rather than a global economic crash. This idea fed the scapegoating of marginalised people through the gaslighting of 'a culture of suspicion' (ibid: 29), allowing the state to simultaneously cut support for marginalised groups whilst claiming to target support on those who truly need it. An ideological ableist rhetoric of the

trustworthy deserving and the deceitful undeserving justified resource deprivation. This ideology shafted disabled people homogenously into a category
of *the vulnerable*, perpetuating a damaging myth. Ryan (2019) also reminds
us that the vulnerability of disabled people is not inevitable but that disabled
people become vulnerable either when they are denied the support they need
or when they have it taken away.

Differently critical (intersectional) disability studies

Critical disability studies are an integral part of the wider discourses of intersectionality. Goodley et al. (2019) problematise how critical disability studies
can become 'all things to all people' (977) and thus lose the potency of their
specificity. However, remaining with the specificity of critical disability studies
might invite exclusivity that loses a relative connectivity to a wider intersectional critical perspective. Schalk and Kim (2020) advocate a 'feminist-of-color
disability method' (38) that contextualises disability in the ideological lega-
cies of wider systemic discriminatory practices and structures that justify the
diversion of resources, such as eugenics, colonialism and welfare reform. The
authors posit that an attention to oppressive ideologies bring to light

> the mutual constitution of ableism, racism, sexism, homophobia, clas-
> sism and cissexism in tracing the raced, gendered, sexual, and classed
> nature of compulsory able-bodiedness and able-mindedness.
>
> (39)

Disability is part of a complex posthuman material-discursive assemblage that
comprises socio-political critical theories and multiple, diverse lived experiences. More recently, critical disability studies have drawn directly from insights from feminist, queer, postcolonial and critical race studies, welcoming
a 'smorgasbord of perspectives' (Goodley et al., 2019: 974). This lived experience cannot be isolated within discrete categories but instead needs to be
located in the mutually constituted power relations of race, gender, class and
sexuality (Schalk & Kim, 2020). In an open letter to the journal *Disability
Studies Quarterly*, 'Radical Disabled Women of Color United,' Miles et al.
(2017) call for critical *intersectional* disability studies in which disability is fully
integrated into a drive for social and political justice for marginalised people.
Meekosha (2011) notes how the European colonisation of the global South
has resulted in poverty and deprivation, yet authors from the global South
tend not to be referenced by those in the North. Power relationships protect
the political and economic interests of the North at the expense of the material
conditions of those in the South. When disability is contextualised in this way,
stories of disability become socially and politically complex.

   Critical disability studies, therefore, is not a separate layer of oppression; it is
integral to the way in which ableist oppression operates in terms of discourses
that underpin ideas of normativity, ability and productivity. The global North

has dominated publications about disability, and there is a danger that these ideas become universalised, rather than being considered as context-specific (Goodley et al., 2019, Meekosha, 2011, Schalk & Kim, 2020). The ways in which we articulate critical theory and our selection of supporting authors, resources and ideas are, themselves, telling of the kinds of knowledge that we privilege and the kinds of assumptions that we make.

As I write this, I hear the radio newsreader state that the impact of this current pandemic is adversely affecting school children, some now behind in their reading, and preschool children, some of whom have not progressed, or have even regressed, in their toilet training. Many learning-disabled people are not literate and are also incontinent, and this anxiety about those who are left behind tells a deeper story of a 'peripheral embodiment' (Mitchel & Snyder, 2015: 7). In the same bulletin, there is a report on the disproportionate level of restraint used on learning-disabled people in NHS mental health hospitals. This is an appalling institutional failure to respond to difference and these news items illustrate deeply embedded discriminatory attitudes towards learning disability.

Differing in conclusions

The experience of disability can be one of marginalisation, disenfranchisement and discrimination, in terms of social, cultural and political participation. A number of discourses enable us to think critically about disability as a phenomenon, including new materialism, posthumanism and intersectionality. These perspectives offer an ecofeminist thinking apparatus that challenges notions of wholeness and coherence and creates new narratives, troubling ideas about humanity as a homogenous group.

As a community dance practitioner, DMP, researcher and educator, I have spent much of my professional life over the past 40 years working with learning-disabled children, young people and adults and their families. Disabled people and their families do not need therapy because of their disability. What creates the need for psychological and emotional support is the distressing impact of discrimination, oppression and lack of opportunities in an ableist world. Goodley et al. (2019) note that we inhabit social, educational and employment landscapes that generate disablism and uphold ableism. For example, they cite the example of school environments as ableist playgrounds, both literally and metaphorically, that reward autonomous and independent learning, whilst calling on a host of 'para-professionals' (987) as specialists to work with disability. However, disability provides an opportunity for all of us to reimagine collective forums, such as the classroom, as places of inclusion, challenging our perception of how we privilege what matters.

In my practising as an ecofeminist DMP practitioner and researcher, I have found critical theories to be essential in helping me understand the dynamic discourses of a range of social identities and the multiple possibilities of their intersections. This process of inquiry is a craft of a lifetime towards evolving a posthuman 'new "we" that expresses the embedded, embodied, relational and affective forces' (Braidotti, 2019: 164–165). *We* are in this together *differently*, and the potential diffractive meeting places of our differences and commonalities support the potential to create new stories about how we live together.

Provocation

How might you locate yourself in terms of social identity?

Map out your own social identity in relation to, for example, age, disability, gender reassignment, marriage and civil partnership, race, religion and belief, sex and sexual orientation, class, mental health status, migrant status, care-experienced young people, those in the criminal justice system, GRT communities and any other social identities that are relevant to you.

What are your personal narratives in relation to these social identities, and how do you relate to concepts of privilege and oppression?

Notes

1 Countertransference refers to the (often) irrational emotional response triggered in the therapist. This process is part of the unconscious dynamics that is created in the emotional field between a therapist and a client.
2 See: www.legislation.gov.uk/ukpga/2010/15/contents
3 For *Disability and Abortion: the Hardest Choice*, see: www.channel4.com/programmes/disability-abortion-the-hardest-choice
4 Diffraction is a term derived from quantum physics (Barad, 2007), and the concept is a useful research tool that enables the mapping of different phenomena across and onto each other to create something new. Diffraction is about convergence, divergence and the multiple possibilities of potential that are created in the collision of things.
5 See David Toole's obituary (Hadoke, 2020): www.theguardian.com/stage/202del0/oct/28/david-toole-obituary
6 NHS is the acronym for the National Health Service in the UK.

References

Andrews, E., Forber-Pratt, A., Mona, L., Lund, E., Pilarski, C. and Balter, R. (2019). #SaytheWord: A disability culture commentary on the erasure of "disability". *Rehabilitation Psychology*, Vol. 64, No. 2, pp. 111–118.

Barad, K. (2007). *Meeting the Universe Halfway: Quantum Physics and the Entanglement of Matter and Meaning*. London: Duke University Press.

Bernard, C. (2022). *Intersectionality for Social Workers: A Practical Introduction to Theory and Practice*. Oxon: Routledge.

Braidotti, R. (2019). *Posthuman Knowledge*. Cambridge: Polity Press.

Crenshaw, K. (1991). Mapping the margins: Intersectionality, identity politics, and violence against women of color. *Stanford Law Review*, Vol. 43, No. 6, pp. 1241–1299.

Frizell, C. (2023a). Bodies, landscapes, and the air that we breathe. *Kritika Kultur*, Vol. 40, pp. 66–73.

Goodley, D., Lawthom, R., Liddiard, K. and Runswick-Cole, K. (2019). Provocations for critical disability studies. *Disability and Society*, Vol. 34, No. 6, pp. 972–997.

Gordy, S. (2020). Champagne, snakes and stealing chips. In S. Salman (ed.), *Made Possible: Stories of Success by People with Learning Disabilities – in Their Own Words*, pp. 55–74. London: Unbound.

Hadoke, T. (2020). David Toole obituary. *The Guardian*, Wednesday 28th October. www.theguardian.com/stage/2020/oct/28/david-toole-obituary

Hickey-Moody, A. (2009). *Unimaginable Bodies: Intellectual Disability, Performance and Becomings*. Rotterdam: Sense Publishers

Liddiard, K., Whitney, S., Evans, K., Watts, L., Vogelmann, E., Spurr, R., Aimes, C., Runswick-Cole, K. and Goodley, D. (2019). Working the edges of posthuman disability studies: Theorising with disabled young people with life-limiting impairments. *Sociology of Health and Illness*, Vol. 41, No. 8, pp. 1473–1487.

Meekosha, H. (2011). Decolonising disability: Thinking and acting globally. *Disability and Society*, Vol. 26, No. 6, pp. 667–682.

Miles, A., Nishida, A. and Forber-Pratt, A. (2017). An open letter to white disability studies and ableist institutions of higher education. *Disability Studies Quarterly*, Vol. 37, No. 3. https://dsq-sds.org/index.php/dsq/article/view/5997/4686

Mitchel, D. and Snyder, S. (2015). *The Biopolitics of Disability: Neoliberalism, Ablenationalism and Peripheral Embodiment*. New York: The University of Michigan Press.

Oliver, M. (1983). *Social Work with Disabled People*. Basingstoke: Macmillan

Ryan, F. (2019). *Crippled: Austerity and the Demonization of Disabled People*. London: Verso.

Schalk, S. and Kim, J. (2020). Integrating race, transforming feminist disability studies. *Signs: Journal of Women in Culture and Society*, Vol. 46, No. 1.

Shakespeare, T. (2013). *Disability Rights and Wrongs Revisited*. Abington: Routledge.

Sinason, V. (2010). *Mental Handicap and the Human Condition: An Analytic Approach to Intellectual Disability*. London: Free Association Books.

Slorach, R. (2016). *A Very Capitalist Condition: A History and Politics of Disability*. London: Bookmarks Publication.

Snow, J. (1994). *What's Really Worth Doing and How to Do It: A Book for People Who Love Someone Labelled Disabled*. Toronto: Inclusion Press.

Thomas, T. (2022). 'Insulting': Shock as NHS uses offensive term for people with learning disability. *The Guardian*, Tuesday 18th October. www.theguardian.com/society/2022/oct/18/insulting-shock-as-nhs-uses-offensive-term-for-people-with-learning-disability?CMP=Share_iOSApp_Other

Ziegler, M. (2020). Disabling language: Why legal terminology should comport with a social model of disability. *Boston College Law Review*, Vol. 61, No. 3, pp. 1182–122.

Interruption 3

Reigniting the dance

It is my mother's birthday. A stroke has confined her to a downstairs bed, too weak to be hoisted into her wheelchair. She has a little movement in her left arm.

I arrive to find her lying still, eyes glazed and unseeing, staring vacantly ahead. Her shallow breath suggests that she is barely clinging on to life. I squeeze her hand and, almost imperceptibly, she squeezes my hand back – a small but unmistakeable response.

I unwrap her present. It feels like a futile game, the gift itself perhaps exposing my desperation to deny our imminent separation. It is a C.D. of Chopin nocturnes that I remember her playing at home decades before on a 45 inch vinyl record to accompany ballet practice.

'Shall I put it on?' I ask, trying to sound upbeat.

I glance out of the window to see that the daffodils are just opening.

Such a pressure to be positive. *How's your mother?* they'd ask. *Oh, about the same*, I would reply, you know – a little weaker each time I visit. I sense their disappointment. It is often a cue to change the subject and I feel a responsibility to shield the world from the disappointment and pain that *things* were not as we desired; *things* would not get better; *things* were not looking up; I cannot uphold the Disney illusion that prosperity and eternal youth lie at our fingertips, if only we could remain positive.

I fiddle with the music centre, fighting back the tears.

Click.

At the press of a button, Chopin's music enters the room.

In an instant, my mother's glazed, unseeing eyes light up. She raises her quivering left arm off the white sheet with a tiny, subtle, but again, unmistakable movement of the hand. A tiny inclination of her head is accompanied by the hint of a song suggested on her out-breath. Just a hint. Or did I imagine it?

Throughout her life, ballet fed and sustained her through difficult times, and now, as she gazes into the gaping mouth of death, the music unwraps

DOI: 10.4324/9781003322658-7

deeply held memories – a re-membering that in dancing she is alive. Her almost-imperceptible-easy-to-miss responses became giant waves in the ocean.

This dance is essential and life-giving in the imminent face of death. My mother's hand rests back on the white sheet in honour of all the mothers, present and past, who bring us into this dance that is life.

4 Dance movement psychotherapy (DMP) through the poetry of ecofeminism

As Maeve arrives, I am struck that we are dressed in identical attire; sky-blue, button-up, long-sleeved shirts and black trousers. I am taken by surprise at my embarrassment at this synchronicity.

On sitting down, Maeve looks at me before shifting her gaze across the studio towards the closed oak doors. I look at her profile, noticing ginger eyebrows framing her blue eyes. Fine hairs cover the pale freckled skin under her cheekbone and her shoulder-length curls sport a hint of orange-red henna. Maeve turns to look at me.

'I was wondering how you do this movement thing.'
'Hmm. It can be hard to move away from the words,' I reply.
'It's very odd. I was excited about coming here to see what it's like to move, if you know what I mean. But now I'm here, it feels terrifying.'

We both look across the empty wooden floor. I am touched by Maeve's expression of vulnerability and her fear of that empty space resonates in me.

'What do you see when you look across the studio?' I ask.
'What do I see?' she repeats, turning back towards me and then looking across the space again. I feel a surge of warmth towards Maeve as she repeats my demand.
'Well, I'm drawn to those cushions at the end.'

Maeve points to the large Turkish carpet cushions that soften the opposite corner of the room.

'We could try sitting over there,' I suggest, surfing the momentum.
'OK,' Maeve says. She does not move.

DOI: 10.4324/9781003322658-8

I sense that I need to continue this momentum in the shift towards movement. I stand up, looking back at Maeve and then slowly walk over to sit on one of the cushions. A voice in my head questions my initiative and I begin to doubt my capacity to hold the anxiety. *Why couldn't I have just waited?* I think. Maeve follows. The cushions scrunch under our weight as we sit side by side, close to the floor. I clasp my hands around my now raised knees and become conscious of my position being perceived as closed. I then cross my feet over, letting my knees drop open and releasing my arms to my sides. Maeve sits stiffly on the cushion next to me, holding tightly onto its edge. She stretches her legs out in front. I am again struck by the synchronicity of our attire. My hands are now resting on the roughly textured cushion cover. I too stretch my legs in front of me, and we turn simultaneously to look at each other. I am silently debating whether I might offer Maeve an invitation into movement. *There is no rush*, I remind myself, refusing a compulsion to make something happen. The look in her eyes is intense. She says nothing. I take in a breath and blurt out,

'We're both dressed the same today.'
'Yes,' she laughs, looking down at her clothes, 'I noticed, but didn't like to say.'
'Hmm,' I nod and smile.
'What do you make of that?'

Maeve raises her eyebrows and looks me up and down. The smile exchanged between us is warm and intimate. There is a light drumming on the roof of the studio as it begins to rain. I look up past the beams into the V-shaped ceiling and then back at Maeve, who is still gazing at me. My intuition invites me to offer Maeve a gentle starting point.

'Would it be helpful if I gave you somewhere to begin with the movement?' I enquire.

Maeve smiles.

'Yes, yes please,' she says.

I reach down to the wooden floor, feeling the cold wood against the palms of my hands. The solid surface is reassuring.

'You could begin standing, or sitting, or . . . feeling your whole body on the floor . . . or . . .'

I leave my sentence in an indeterminate state. Leaning forwards, I push my hands into the floor, allowing my elbows to bend, and then push myself back up, bringing my hands to my knees. We look towards the empty space, hovering on the cusp of a liminal space. Maeve tentatively leans forwards to put the palms of her hands on the floor and she looks around the room. She brings her hands back to either side of her hips and pushes them into the cushion, sliding off feet first and rolling onto her back about a metre away from me. She stretches her arms out sideways, opening her fingers to flatten the palms of her hands on the floor. Slowly she turns her head towards me. We look at each other again. The drumming of the rain intensifies.

'Perhaps take a breath and focus on the different parts of your body in contact with the floor,' I say. I notice a small woodlouse making its way under the radiator.

Maeve begins to curve her spine slowly on the floor, stretching through her arms and legs.

'I really want to roll across the floor,' she says.

'Mm,' I resist the temptation to offer permission.

Maeve moves her arms over her head, to create a long line from her fingers to her toes, and she begins to roll slowly and sequentially to the centre of the studio, as if caressing the floor indulgently with shifting surfaces of her body. Repeating the roll for a third time, she pauses on her stomach, face down towards the wooden floor, where she stays very still. I am captivated. Maeve makes a pattering sound with her fingertips on the floorboards, echoing the rain that continues to drum on the roof. She stops. The rain continues. She pulls her elbows in under her body, curving her spine, and places her hands on the floor under her shoulders to push her weight back onto her knees. Tucking her toes under her feet, she continues to push herself up to standing. She opens her arms to the side and slides her right foot along the floor as if skating in slow motion. She pushes through the air with the palms of her hands travelling across the floor and continues pushing forwards, right and left, stopping at the wall and turning to face the studio space. Maeve looks at me momentarily, slowly scans the room and then looks back at me.

The rain subsides and then stops. The silence is punctuated by the gentle ticking of the clock, and we continue to look at each other.

I stand, slowly. Together, we wander back to the red velvet chairs. I glance at the clock. We still have some time. We sit silently, my gaze focused downwards.

Maeve cuts through the silence.

'It's strange how hard it is to fill the space without being told what to do, but once I began, I just let my movement take over.'

Dancing between modalities

As I recall this encounter with Maeve, I am reminded of how it can seem very unfamiliar and sometimes awkward to shift from a space of experiencing and thinking about the world through language into a space of generating new relational and emotional discoveries through improvised movement. The vignette presented here was a few sessions into the process and we were still finding a way to work together. Maeve had had previous experience of verbal therapy and was now interested in *how you do this movement thing*. This vignette is an example of how I supported Maeve to claim the movement space, as we navigated a delicate and intimate exchange. The synchronicity of being dressed in identical attire somehow brought my vulnerability to the surface and this was a useful reminder of the fragility of the encounter that we were stepping into together.

Had you been the practitioner, the relational assemblage would have shaped a differently emerging encounter. I wonder about your experience of shifting between language and moving bodies or other art forms in which rational language is not the primary means of expression. In the dance world, a culture is created in which creatively moving bodies become a normalised mode of expression; however, outside of the specificity of that professional field, language can become a dominant mode of relating and making sense of the world. Indoor spaces tend to be filled with stuff, such as furniture, unless it is a specifically designated movement space, inadvertently prohibiting the potential for movement. In facilitating working indoors, such as in client work, supervision or when teaching, I try to create spaces that offer implicit invitations to engage creatively. For example, in my private practice, which is the context for Maeve's process, I have a small studio space that was originally a fifteenth-century barn. I deliberately leave the centre of the space clear as an implicit invitation for moving bodies. At one end, art materials are available and around the space, an array of mats, stretch cloths and other materials are suggestive of movement and play. I have one or two drums, including a djembe that I sometimes use as accompaniment. In addition, I have stones, shells, driftwood and other things that I have borrowed from outdoor places, always on loan and to be returned one day. These borrowed things bring an awareness of the outdoors inside, providing material reminders of the earth as our home. Overall, the materiality of the context invites creativity. I also work outside, usually on moorlands, where the environment is less predictable, in terms of fluctuating weather, seasonal change and the cycles of growth of fauna and flora. In Chapter 5, I will be further discussing the potential of working outdoors.

Maeve came to me for DMP *because* of the potential for movement; yet, even though we shared that intention, there was initially an unfamiliarity and awkwardness in trusting the vital intelligence of the improvising moving body to take her into new territories. That moment of transition from engaging through language into the materiality of the moving body, and back again,

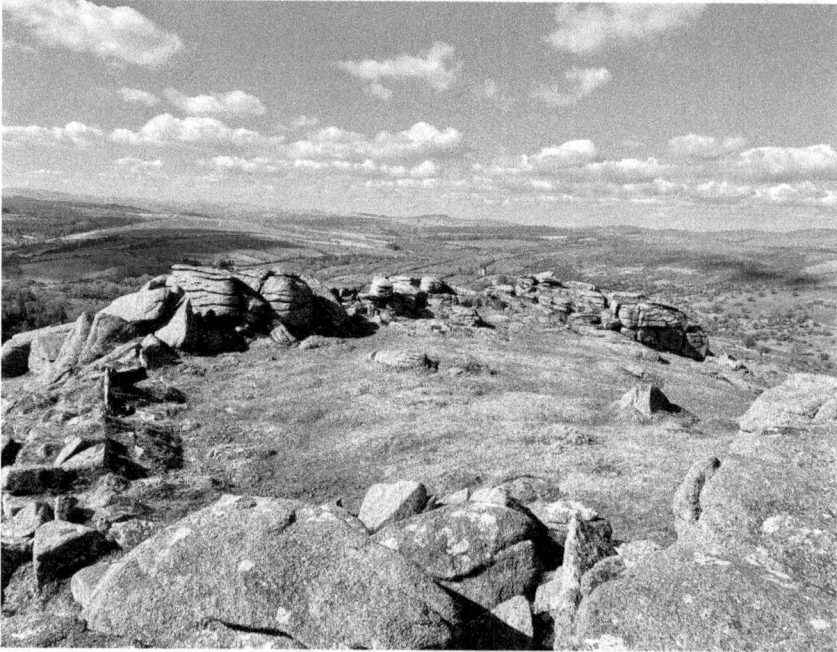

Figure 4.1 Dartmoor outdoor working space.
Source: Photograph by the author.

harbours a Cartesian[1] dualism that subordinates the wisdom of bodies against the perceived superior wisdom of the rational mind through deeply embedded white Eurocentric social, cultural and political inscriptions. These are complex waters of matter and discourse through which bodies swim. Maeve observed the gap between the idea and the reality: the disconnect between her excitement in embarking on a therapeutic process that makes space for improvising bodies and the terror induced by confronting the reality of that potential. Maeve was inhabiting a menopausal, female body with historical experiences, for example, of being a migrant. I later discovered that she had also suffered abusive relationships within the context of patriarchal discourses that privilege able-bodied, male, affluent, well-educated, heteronormative, white European embodiments of the human, as represented in by Leonardo da Vinci's *Vitruvian Man*[2] (Braidotti, 2022).

Potent discourses hover in moments of hesitation. In the transference, I came to represent figures of authority and oppression for Maeve and this became the pivotal place in our work together. At times, I struggled with feelings of vulnerability and inadequacy in the relational field, whilst simultaneously realising that Maeve was experiencing me as a powerful and dominant force. This was a complex intra-active, material-discursive space of poetic emergence.

Dancing bodies as material-discursive poetry

Material-discursive bodies-in-movement create and are created by a poetic language of dance, through which we understand and locate ourselves as part of
the wider poetry of ecologies of diversely moving bodies. This kinaesthetic
leaning into the corporeality of relational matter is grounded in contingent
practices of doing, emerging and becoming. Bodies unfold together with
other bodies of all kin(ds) within relational and affective matrices that are
materially and discursively situated. Dance is a way of understanding this intra-
active emergence, as we repeatedly bring ourselves into relational alignment
with a sentient, moving world. This material entanglement, however, is also
discursively implicated with social, cultural and political inscriptions. Notions
of bodies as biological matter(s) become entangled with notions of bodies as
manifestations of ideological, social, political and cultural constructs, to such
a degree that the possibility of unconstructed materiality comes into question
(Butler, 2011).

As discussed in Chapter 3, dynamic intra-active material bodies-in-movement
are always the body politic. Take, for example, female bodies, disabled bodies,
queer bodies, racialised bodies, older bodies, other-than-human bodies and all
the other bodies that have been subordinated, oppressed and othered within
powerful discourses. These social and environmental categories are themselves
diverse in membership. For instance, the female body has many manifestations
and intersections. In the film *Isadora's Children*,[3] three women, in three very
different bodies, are impacted in different ways by loss in relation to Isadora
Duncan's choreography created following the tragic loss of her children in an
accident. The film follows a young, white, able-bodied dance student as she
studies the choreography of the dance, whilst also trying to understand the
complex emotional content of a story of loss. The second woman, a white-
skinned dancer with Down's syndrome, is rehearsing to perform the part of
Isadora, moving sensitively into the role. The third woman, an older black
woman with restricted mobility and who walks with a stick, attends this performance. She returns home to her flat alone and lights an incense stick in
honour of her dead son. As she gets ready for bed, she closes the curtain and
begins to improvise her own poignant dance of loss. The film offers powerful
images of different ways that female bodies can be inhabited, each with their
own unique expression. Thematically, loss is pivotal in the film, and the expression of the moving bodies is equal to (if not taking precedence over) dialogic
language.

The body politic is a place of performativity. Bodies are never just bodies.
Manning (2014) proposes that '(a) philosophy of the body never begins with
the body: it *bodies*' (163), preferring body as a verb (to body) rather than as
a noun (a body). This processual idea of what bodies do cuts across Cartesian binaries, as bodying processes affect and are affected within ecologies of
movement. Manning (2012) describes how '(i)nfants bathe in pure experience' (10) through this bodying. Moving, sensing, feeling bodies are central

to discovering and making sense of the world through improvisation, play and experimentation, dancing through liminal gaps and articulating new connections between ideas and experience.

Thus, embodied ways of knowing are immersed in the idea of *knowing* as living in the world empathically and creatively. This is different from an idealised, romanticised and grandiose idea of bodies as inherently *all-knowing* (as if there is such a thing). Bodies are inherently entangled in cultural, social and political constructs and discourses that cannot be separated as discrete silos of embodied *knowing*. Bodies are material-discursive processes that are creating and created by the world again and again. As I write this, I am aware that there is no linear path of understanding and ask you (again) to stay with the trouble of being with processes that elide distinct and tidy definitions. These riddles are provocations that lead us deeper into enigmatic landscapes of diverse material-discursive bodies, rather than opening doors to tidy definitions. Again, language as the representative tool to hand falls short of its capacity to become the experience of a body; however, I will try to articulate some ideas that give this kind of knowledge some watery shape.

Neimans (2019) reminds us that we are primarily 'watery bodies in a watery world' (65) and that this matter of our wateriness is a 'wellspring for new ontological and ethical paradigms' (7). We bathe, literally and metaphorically, in the waters of experience through dance and it is perhaps no coincidence that DMP practitioners arguably lead the way into new currents and tributaries of ethico-onto-epistemologies in these turbulent waters – those currents and tributaries being ethical attitudes of care that are embedded in diverse ways of experiencing and of knowing the world. Intra-active bodies-in-movement are orienting catalysts for relational experiences as part of wider watery processes of life. I become conscious of encountering the materiality of the world, not in a search for some notion of an underlying truth but more in a quest for the knowledge of what might be possible in my ever-changing 'sensory-kinetic palette of possibilities' (LaMothe, 2015: 57). Moving bodies signal our arrival into existence, as sperms race towards eggs in flurries of activity. Cells divide to become foetuses, participating in 'the process of becoming itself' (LaMothe, 2015: 90). We join the world through dances of fleshy, visceral bodies that unfold as the raw material of existence. As a DMP practitioner, researcher and educator, the poetry of ecofeminism embeds the notion of subjectivity in material-discursive bodies-in-movement as affective flows within assemblages of many different forms of life.

The creativity of moving bodies provides a place of potential empathic reconnection with the ecology. In her research into kinaesthetic empathy, Rova (2017) asserts that when we cut off from our bodily empathetic capacity, we can become desensitised to that affective participation within a relational ecology. She cites an example of working with a nursery nurse, who recalls her response to a patient's violent behaviour. In a subsequent reflective practice session, the nurse is confronted by the somatic impact of this incident, noting 'how traumatic work experiences often caused her to disconnect from her body in order to "get through" her shift' (ibid: 171). This example of how we can disconnect from our empathic connection so that we can *get through the shift* (aka life) poses broader ethical issues of becoming desensitised to a normalised violence that disconnects us from the intra-active field of kinship. This disconnection from our kinaesthetic empathic relationship with the world around us invites the insidious violence of un-care, entitlement and exceptionalism (Weintrobe, 2013).

Dance as poetry in therapeutic practice

In the UK (at the point of writing this book), DMP, like the other arts therapies and psychotherapy, is not a protected title. Practitioners train (rigorously) at the masters' level in DMP and licensed practitioners use various descriptors in their professional titles, including dance, movement, non-stylised movement, environmental movement, somatic practice, expressive arts, body, embodied and more, along with the words therapy and psychotherapy, to underscore the kind of practice offered.

The differentiation and connection between movement and dance is, indeed, an old chestnut. Both words are present in the graduating title, dance movement psychotherapy, without a conjunction (i.e., and, or), unhyphenated (i.e., no connecting dash) and without punctuation (i.e., no comma between the two words) and one might infer that the two words are synonymous. Some practitioners will suggest that the word dance might be misleading, given public perceptions of what dance *is*; however, others emphasise that dance, as an art form, is central to their practice. I wonder how you, the reader, navigate these waters in your understanding of the title both semantically and in practice. The distinction between movement and dance might arguably be a sematic issue of the representational nature of language. That is, the language we use can only be a representation of the thing we describe, rather than the thing itself.

LaMothe (2015, 2020) develops a philosophy of bodily becoming, in which she claims dance as an ethical art form that is 'vital for our humanity' (LaMothe, 2015: 3). We evolve a way of knowing the world through our capacity for kinetic awareness and this knowledge arises from a place of kinaesthetic sensing, feeling and being present to moment-to-moment (em)bodied encounters. Thus, bodied ways of knowing (aka dance) are grounded in *knowing* as living in the world poetically. The boundary between non-stylised moving processes and the art of dance is blurred and gives rise to rich ethical, ontological, epistemological, political and aesthetic questions in dance discourses, as were developed, for example, by the postmodern dance makers of the 1960s and 1970s. The postmodern dance era took a diversion from traditional creative and aesthetic principles that had shaped dance performance and played with the blurring of boundaries between movement as a stylised art form and the potential of pedestrian, everyday movement as dance.

This place of knowing emanates from the immediate lived kinetic experience that can be thought about through improvisational movement (Fraleigh,

2019, Sheets-Johnstone, 2011). The liminal space of relational improvisation fosters 'a return to the wonder of lived embodied experiences in the present moment' (Barbour, 2018: 242). The place of improvisation is the place where 'things draw apart, alternate, disintegrate, or assemble throughout a creative whole' (Frahleigh, 2019: 65). This is the place of responsiveness to the improvisation of the world. It is always relational and situated within intra-active spaces in which all material things have an agentic capacity (as discussed in Chapter 2). Improvisational movement can put us in touch with our empathic capacity, thus bringing us into an emotional relationship with the world. I remember running a workshop for chaplains at a conference on death and dying. An older woman in the group, who claimed never to have danced before, found a fluidity in her body that was beautiful and deeply moving. As she moved, she lifted her arms to the sky and tears poured down her face. She had realised, she said, as if for the first time, just how much she loved the aesthetic beauty of the earth. She said,

> *I suddenly feel so sad at the realisation that when I die, I will no longer see, smell, hear, taste and touch this beautiful earth.*

Maeve entered her improvisational moving body, arriving relationally into the material world around her, with me as therapist by her side. For example, the surfaces of her body came into conversation with the wooden floor, the smooth velvet chair cover, the roughly textured Turkish carpet cushions and the sound of rain drumming on the roof. This tending towards the bodily self (Ahmed, 2010, Manning, 2012) is a place of encounter. Maeve entered the therapy space wondering how to do *this movement thing*. She had an intuitive drive to move away from the words and enter a bodily knowing through movement, yet the reality was that this was an unfamiliar territory that lay beyond a normative threshold.

Dance movement psychotherapy as a profession: poetic diffractions

DMP practitioners in the West follow in the footsteps of the documented practice of Marion Chase, who, in the 1940s, initiated the use of dance to facilitate a therapeutic process with psychiatric patients in the US (Sandel & Chaiklin, 1993). Since that time, DMP has borrowed from psychotherapeutic paradigms to find its rhizomatic becoming. In an arts therapy survey, Zubala and Karkou (2015) identified that preferred approaches of DMP practitioners (i.e., of those practitioners who were interviewed) included humanistic and object relations reference points and in particular, attachment and Winnicottian theories. A number of psychotherapeutic theoretical models have underpinned DMP practice, for example, humanistic (Fisher, 2017, Meekums, 2002), gestalt (Feldman, 2016), psychoanalytic (Bloom, 2006, Penfield, 2001, Siegal, 1984), Jungian (Goldhahn, 2015, 2022, Pallaro, 1999), post-Jungian

(Bacon, 2020) and transpersonal (Hayes, 2007, 2013). Practices have evolved, such as Authentic Movement (Bacon, 2010, 2017, 2020, Goldhahn, 2015, 2022, Pallaro, 1999), and Goldhahn (2022) explores Authentic Movement as both a practice and a research method supporting a spirit of creativity in the wider field of arts and arts therapies. Additionally, environmental movement has evolved as a practice (Frizell, 2014, 2020, Frizell & Poynor, 2023, Poynor, 2018, 2023, Reeve, 2011) and as more recent ecofeminist, posthuman and new materialist practices (Allegranti & Silas, 2021, Allegranti, 2019, Frizell, 2020, 2021a, 2023c, 2023a, 2023b).

In 2008, the professional association in the UK made a formal shift from the term dance movement *therapy* (DMT) to dance movement *psychotherapy*. I remember that this shift was not without its contentions. Although a majority of members of the association voted to change the name to the *Association for Dance Movement Psychotherapy* (ADMPUK), there was a significant minority voice that did not consider the new name to be an accurate representation of their practice. One of the arguments for introducing the word *psychotherapy* was to align the profession to psychotherapeutic practices, rather than medical healthcare therapies, such as physiotherapy and occupational therapy. Another powerful subtext was the alignment to psychotherapy as a more familiar talking cure and language-based intervention and its associated professional power relations. For DMP practitioners, this debate was about professional identity politics, in relation to the pervasive hierarchies of professional worth, in a climate of Western neoliberalism and advanced capitalism. As DMP practitioners, we (although *we* are hardly a homogenous group) perhaps get trapped in the liminal spaces of professional identity politics.

DMP practitioners from this wide range of approaches have typically worked with voices that have been subjugated within dominant discourses; that is, voices of peoples who are vulnerable to being othered, for example, patients in acute psychiatry (Rova & Behm, 2023, Stanton-Jones, 1992), people with refugee and migrant status (Aranda et al., 2020, Rova et al., 2020, Singer, 2017), learning-disabled people (Barjacoba-Souto, 2023, Curtis, 2017, Frizell, 2012, 2014, 2017, 2021, Unkovich et al., 2017), care-experienced young people (Ballal, 2023), people with early onset dementia (Allegranti, 2021), patients within prisons and medium secure units (Ballal, 2023, Batcup, 2013, 2023, Law, 2023, Ramasubramanian & Batcup, 2021) and many more.

There are also practitioners who work within the interface of DMP and other arts practices, for example, Diener's (2023) work with disabled children, young people and their families in which she brings the principles of DMP and dance performance into building community; Allegranti's (2021) work that brings together DMP, choreographic research practice and activism with individuals and families affected by young onset dementia; and Steinmuller (2023) who combines her skills as a DMP, as a teacher and as a performer in her work creating performance with and by young people who experience mental health issues.

DMP practice and research in the UK have unfolded as a mercurial and multifaceted profession that continues to shapeshift through material-discursive spaces. It has evolved through rhizomatic processes that span, for example, healthcare, community care, social care, the voluntary sector, education, the criminal justice system and private practice, transforming across psychotherapeutic paradigms. There is no one history of DMP; rather, there is an assemblage of professional researching and practising that has evolved, some of which is documented in publications, whereby practitioners and researchers have taken authorship of their ideas and much more that has developed without the published visibility that they might deserve. Hence, Eberhard-Kaechele (2017) calls for DMP practitioners to 'get out your laptops!' (245) lest the innovative ideas that are the mainstay of DMP practitioners are inadvertently appropriated by researchers and clinicians with a stronger professional visibility (for example, verbal psychotherapy) who discover moving bodies (their own and those of their clients) in clinical practice rooms.

DMP is a lesser-known profession, and DMP practitioners and researchers repeatedly become pioneers within professional landscapes that are cautious of the unfamiliar. This is particularly the case within the unstable economic climates of a neoliberalist ideology that brings with it a culture of hyper-rationality, marketisation and managerialism to the delivery of public services. This role as pioneer can be a lonely place and there are times when DMP, as a diverse professional collective, has seemed to lose its way in a desire to define a pre-existing entity (Eberhard-Kaechele, 2017, Lemon Williams, 2019, Meekums, 2014, Vulcan, 2013). Yet this eclectic identity is also a strength.

Dancing poetic in conclusions

Overall, DMP is an eclectic profession that draws on a wide theoretical range and comes in many shapes and forms. The connecting thread between these differing approaches, methods and philosophies is a commitment to the entanglement of relational moving bodies as a catalyst for fostering well-being. I remind myself of this as I step away from my desk and stand, feet apart, arms dropped by my side.

The soles of my feet converse with the roughly textured carpet. A car alarm begins outside in a kind of relentless repetition. It stops. My left hand lifts slowly towards my face and I feel my cold fingertips against my skin. My right arm reaches sideways and I stretch towards it, curving my spine and shifting my weight between my feet to steady myself. I begin to sink towards the floor but find myself, at the same time, reaching upwards. A blackbird sings outside the window and my movement becomes fluid as I twist towards that song, finding an energy that meets with each mo(ve)ment before it disappears.

This chapter has located DMP within some of the discourses about moving, dancing bodies in and as psychotherapy, offering the ways in which ecofeminist, new materialist, posthuman thinking can help shape the philosophical principles of practice and research. This profession of DMP can be perceived

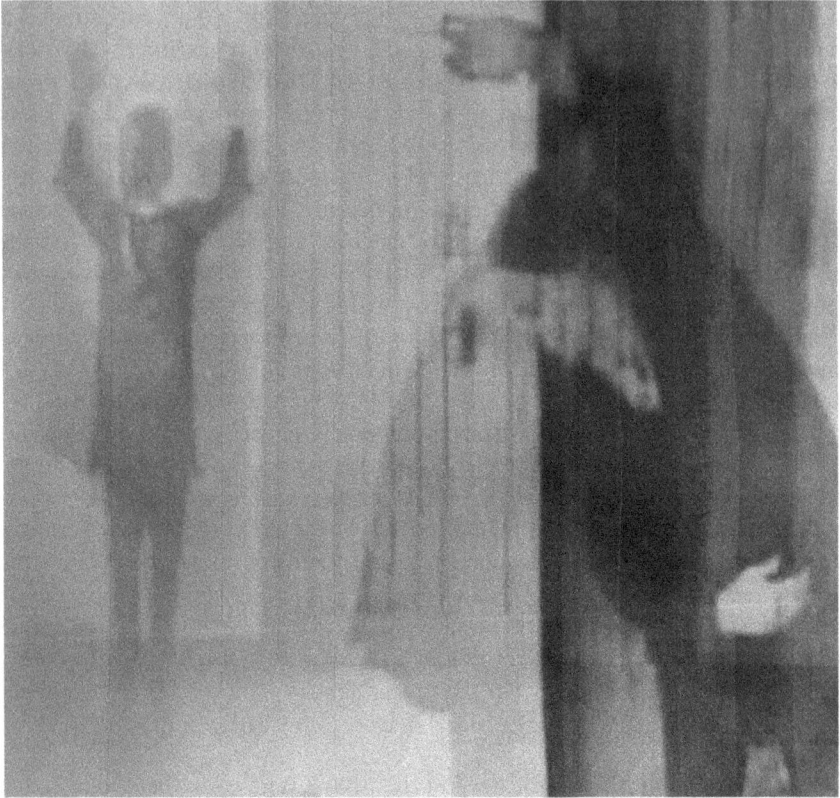

Figure 4.2 Material bodies.
Source: Photograph by the author.

(and at times perceives itself) as elusive, indeterminate, niche and highly specialised. It also carries a breadth of accessibility in its potential to soften the focus on language, as material modes of relational bodied expression are invited into the light.

I began this chapter illustrating one of those moments of transition from words into movement in my work with Maeve. Reflecting on that mo(ve)ment invites discussion about the privileging of language and discourse over the materiality of intra-active movement practice. Improvising bodies are nomadic and processual, inhabiting (and being inhabited by) the unpredictability and conjunctive nature of moving through the world experientially. The corporeality of bodies as relational matter(s) is always situated discursively, with the personal and the political entangled and mutually implicated. We simultaneously create and are created by identity politics and pervasive social categories. DMP has developed its own ethico-onto-epistemology of moving bodies, as well as borrowing from and diffracting with(in) psychotherapeutic paradigms. The conscious awareness of movement that is already going on and that awaits discovery in those ongoing points of diffraction turns me towards lived experience, immersive intra-action and immanence. Material bodies are created *as* movement, and that poetry continues from our conception until our last breath.

Provocation

Settle somewhere either indoors or outdoors. Soften the focus of your vision. Move into your senses and allow your movement to arrive into the materiality of the world. Simply allow that movement to lead you somewhere, somehow.

Find a pen and paper and give the pen permission to intra-act in any way that seems fit.

Where did this invitation take you?

Notes

1 Cartesian refers to the philosophy of René Descartes that separated the thinking, rational mind from the visceral, moving body.
2 Leonardo da Vinci's drawing of the Vitruvian Man representing the ideally proportioned man.
3 *Isadora's Children* is a film directed by Damien Manivel. See trailer here: www.youtube.com/watch?v=L7foZbI1ZIE

References

Ahmed, S. (2010). Orientations matter. In D. Coole and S. Frost (eds.), *New Materialisms: Ontology, Agency and Politics*, pp. 234–257. London: Duke University Press.

Allegranti, B. (2019). Moving kinship: Between choreography, performance and the more-than-human. In S. Prickett and H. Thomas (eds.), *The Routledge Handbook for Dance Studies*. London: Routledge.

Allegranti, B. (2021). Dancing Activism. In H. Wengrower and S. Chaiklin (eds.), *Dance and Creativity within Dance Movement Therapy. International Perspectives*, pp. 157–177. New York/Oxon: Routledge.

Allegranti, B. and Silas, J. (2021). Intra-active signatures in Capoeira: More-than-human pathways towards activism. *Emotion, Space and Society*, Vol. 38, pp. 1–11.

Aranda, E., Hills de Zárate, M. and Panhofer, H. (2020). Transformed ground, transformed body: Clinical implications for dance movement therapy with forced migrants. *Body, Movement and Dance in Psychotherapy: An International Journal for Theory, Research and Practice*, Vol. 15, No. 3, pp. 156–170.

Bacon, J. (2010). The voice of her body: Somatic practices as a basis for creative research methodology. *Journal of Dance and Somatic Practices*, Vol. 2, No. 1, pp. 63–74.

Bacon, J. (2017). Authentic Movement as a Practice for Wellbeing. In V. Karkou, S. Oliver and S. Lycouris (eds.), *The Oxford Handbook of Dance and Wellbeing*, pp. 149–164. Oxford: Oxford University Press.

Bacon, J. (2020). Informed by the goddess: Explicating a processual methodology. In A. Williamson and B. Sellers-Young (eds.), *Spiritual Herstories: Call of the Soul in Dance Research*, pp. 69–87. Bristol: Intellect.

Ballal, A. (2023). Dancing in the kitchen; using creativity and embodiment to promote a decolonising approach to psychotherapy. In C. Frizell and M. Rova (eds.), *Creative Bodies in Therapy, Performance and Community Research and Practice that Brings Us Home*, pp. 131–142. London: Routledge.

Barbour, K. (2018). Dancing epistemology. Situating feminist analysis. In S. Fraleigh (ed.), *Back to the Dance Itself: Phenomenologies of the Body in Performance*, pp. 233–246. California, CA: Illinois.

Barjacoba-Souto, B. (2023). Dancing with Stephen: Reconnecting with the body in a search for closure. In C. Frizell and M. Rova (eds.), *Creative Bodies in Therapy, Performance and Community Research and Practice that Brings Us Home*, pp. 171–179. London: Routledge.

Batcup, D. (2013). A Discussion of the dance movement psychotherapy literature relative to prisons and medium secure units. *Body, Movement and Dance in Psychotherapy: An International Journal for Theory, Research and Practice*, Vol. 8, No. 1, pp. 5–16.

Batcup, D. (2023). Indominus Rex; Developing mentalisation with offenders through externalisation and creativity in a dance movement psychotherapy group. In C. Frizell and M. Rova (eds.), *Creative Bodies in Therapy, Performance and Community Research and Practice that Brings Us Home*, pp. 162–170. London: Routledge.

Bloom, K. (2006). *The Embodied Self: Movement and Psychoanalysis*. London: Karnac.

Braidotti, R. (2022). *Posthuman Feminism*. Cambridge: Polity Press.

Butler, J. (2011). *Bodies that Matter*. New York: Routledge.

Curtis, S. (2017). On becoming a monkey. In G. Unkovich, C. Butte and J. Butler (eds.), *Dance Movement Psychotherapy with People with Learning Disabilities*, pp. 81–93. Oxon: Routledge.

Diener, J. (2023). Finding my way home; An embodied journey to building and inclusive dance community. In C. Frizell and M. Rova (eds.), *Creative Bodies in Therapy, Performance and Community: Research and Practice that Brings Us Home*, pp. 122–130. London: Routledge.

Eberhard-Kaechele, M. (2017). A political perspective on dance movement psychotherapy on interdisciplinary pathways: Are we finding or losing our way? *Body, Movement and Dance in Psychotherapy: An International Journal for Theory, Research and Practice*, Vol. 12, No. 4, pp. 237–251.

Feldman, Y. (2016). How body psychotherapy Influenced me to become a dance movement psychotherapist. *Body, Movement and Dance in Psychotherapy: An International Journal for Theory, Research and Practice*, Vol. 11, Nos. 2–3, pp. 103–113.

Fisher, P. (2017). The recovery journey: The place and value of dance movement psychotherapy with clients with alcohol or substance misuse. In H. Payne (ed.), *Essentials of Dance Movement Psychotherapy: International Perspectives on Theory, Research, and Practice*, pp. 223–236. London: Routledge.

Fraleigh, S. (2019). A philosophy of the improvisational body. In L. Midgelow (ed.), *The Oxford Handbook of Improvisation in Dance*, pp. 65–88. New York: Oxford University Press.

Frizell, C. (2012). Embodiment and the supervisory task. *Body, Movement and Dance in Psychotherapy: An International Journal for Theory, Research and Practice*, Vol. 7, No. 4, pp. 293–304.

Frizell, C. (2014). Discovering the language of the ecological body. *Self and Society: An International Journal for Humanistic Psychology*, Vol. 41, No. 4, pp. 15–21.

Frizell, C. (2017). Entering the world: Dance movement psychotherapy and the complexity of beginnings with learning disabled clients. In G. Unkovich, C. Buttee and J. Butler (eds.), *Dance Movement Psychotherapy with People with Learning Disabilities: Out of the Shadows, into the Light*, pp. 9–21. Abingdon: Routledge.

Frizell, C. (2020). Reclaiming our innate vitality: Bringing embodied narratives to life through dance movement psychotherapy. In A. Williamson and B. Sellers-Young (eds.), *Spiritual Herstories: Call of the Soul in Dance Research*, pp. 207–220. Bristol: Intellect.

Frizell, C. (2021a). *Towards Posthuman Dancing Subjects: A Critical Commentary Assemblage that Interrupts Five Published Works through the Lens of Practice-led, New Materialist Research*. Unpublished thesis. London: Goldsmiths, University of London.

Frizell, C. (2021b). Learning disability imagined differently: An evaluation of interviews with parents about discovering that their child has Down's syndrome. *Disability and Society*, Vol. 36, No. 10, pp. 1574–1593.

Frizell, C. (2023a). Bodies, landscapes, and the air that we breathe. *Kritika Kultur*, Vol. 40, pp. 66–73.

Frizell, C. (2023b). Coming home to a posthuman body; Finding hopefulness in those who care. In D. Parker, C. Jackson and L. Aspey (eds.), *Holding the Hope: Reviving/restoring Psychological and Spiritual Agency in the Face of Climate Change*, pp. 76–85. Monmouth: PCCS Books.

Frizell, C. (2023c). The cat, the foal and other meetings that make a difference: Posthuman research that re-animates our responsiveness to knowing and becoming. In C. Frizell and M. Rova (eds.), *Creative Bodies in Therapy, Performance and Community Research and Practice that Brings Us Home*, pp. 50–61. London: Routledge.

Frizell, C. and Poynor, H. (2023). The matriarch and the mollusc and all things in between. In C. Frizell and M. Rova (eds.), *Creative Bodies in Therapy, Performance and Community Research and Practice that Brings Us Home*, pp. 180–190. London: Routledge.

Goldhahn, E. (2015). Towards a new ontology and name for 'Authentic Movement'. *Journal of Dance and Somatic Practices*, Vol. 7, No. 2, pp. 273–285.

Goldhahn, E. (2022). *Reflections on Authentic Movement; Theory, Practice and Arts-led Research*. Oxon: Routledge.

Hayes, J. (2007). *Performing the Dreams of Your Body; Plays of Animation and Compassion*. Chichester: Archive Publishing.

Hayes, J. (2013). *Soul and Spirit in Dance Movement Psychotherapy: A Transpersonal Approach*. London: Jessica Kingsley.

LaMothe, K. (2015). *Why We Dance: A Philosophy of Bodily Becoming*. New York: Columbia University Press.

LaMothe, K. (2020). Writing why we dance: The predicament, pitfalls, potential and promise of writing about dance and spirituality. In A. Williamson and B. Sellers-Young (eds.), *Spiritual Herstories: Call of the Soul in Dance Research*, pp. 393–413. Bristol: Intellect.

Law, A. (2023). Sing your way home; Designing a creative group intervention in the women's prison as a dance movement therapist in Singapore. In C. Frizell and M. Rova (eds.), *Creative Bodies in Therapy, Performance and Community Research and Practice that Brings Us Home*, pp. 143–151. London: Routledge.

Lemon Williams, J. (2019). (Re-)defining dance/movement therapy fifty years hence. *American Journal of Dance Therapy*, Vol. 41, pp. 273–285.

Manning, E. (2012). *Always More than One: Individuation's Dance*. Durham: Duke University Press.

Manning, E. (2014). Wondering the world directly – or, how movement outruns the subject. *Body and Society*, Vol. 20, Nos. 3–4, pp. 162–188.

Meekums, B. (2002). *Dance Movement Therapy*. London: Sage.

Meekums, B. (2014). Becoming visible as a profession in a climate of competitiveness: The role of research. *Body, Movement and Dance in Psychotherapy: An International Journal for Theory, Research and Practice*, Vol. 9, No. 3, pp. 123–137.

Neimans, A. (2019). *Bodies of Water*. New York: Bloomsbury.

Pallaro, P. (ed.). (1999). *Authentic Movement: Essays by Mary Starks Whitehouse, Janet Adler and Joan Chodorow*. London: Jessica Kingsley.

Penfield, K (2001). Movement as a way to the unconscious. In Y. Searle and I. Streng (eds.), *Where Analysis Meets the Arts: The Integration of Arts Therapies with Psychoanalysis*, pp. 107–126. London: Karnac.

Poynor, H. (2018). Earth, Tree, Rock and Sea. *Journal of Dance and Somatic Practices*, Vol. 10, No. 2, pp. 169–173.

Poynor, H. (2023). Is that yoga or are you just making it up?. In C. Frizell and M. Rova (eds.), *Creative Bodies in Therapy, Performance and Community Research and Practice that Brings Us Home*, pp. 101–108. London: Routledge.

Ramasubramanian, P. and Batcup, D. (2021). Exploring maternal and erotic transference in DMP with a sex offender. In S. Hastilow and M. Leibmann (eds.), *Arts Therapies and Sexual Offending*, pp. 79–96. London: Jessica Kingsley.

Reeve, S. (2011). *Nine Ways of Seeing a Body*. Axminster: Triarchy Press.

Rova, M. (2017). Embodying kinaesthetic empathy through interdisciplinary practice-based research. *The Arts in Psychotherapy*, Vol. 55, pp. 164–173.

Rova, M. and Behm, M. (2023). *Borderlands: Exploring creativity as a practice of liminality in the arts therapies*. In C. Frizell and M. Rova (eds.), *Creative Bodies in Therapy, Performance and Community Research and Practice that Brings Us Home*, pp. 152–161. Oxon: Routledge.

Rova, M., Burrell, C. and Cohen, M. (2020). Existing in-between two worlds: Supporting asylum seeking women living in temporary accommodation through a creative movement and art intervention. *Body, Movement and Dance in Psychotherapy: An International Journal for Theory, Research and Practice*, Vol. 15, No. 3, pp. 204–218.

Sandel, S. and Chaiklin, S. (eds.). (1993). *Foundations of Dance Movement Therapy: The Life and Work of Marion Chace*. Columbia Maryland: The Marion Chace Memorial Fund ADTA.

Sheets-Johnstone, M. (2011). *The Primacy of Movement*. Philadelphia: John Benjamins Pub. Co.

Siegal, E. (1984). *Dance Movement Therapy: Mirror of Ourselves. The Psychoanalytic Approach*. New York: Human Sciences Press.

Singer, A. (2017). Building relations: A methodological consideration of dance and wellbeing in psychosocial work with war-affected refugee children and their families. In V. Karkou, S. Oliver and S. Lycouris (eds.), *The Oxford Handbook of Dance and Wellbeing*. Oxford: Oxford University Press.

Stanton-Jones, K. (1992). *An Introduction to Dance Movement Therapy in Psychiatry*. London: Routledge.

Steinmuller, E. (2023). Lives transformed through dance: The art of dance as a catalyst for personal transformation. In C. Frizell and M. Rova (eds), *Creative Bodies in Therapy, Performance and Community: Research and Practice that Brings Us Home*, pp. 76–86. Oxon: Routledge.

Unkovich, G., Butté, C. and Butler, J. (eds.). (2017). *Dance Movement Psychotherapy with People with Learning Disabilities: Out of the Shadows, into the Light*. Abingdon: Routledge.

Vulcan, M. (2013). Crossing the somatic–semiotic divide: The troubled question of Dance/Movement Therapists (DMTs) professional identity. *The Arts in Psychotherapy*, Vol. 40, No. 1, pp. 6–19.

Weintrobe, S. (ed.). (2013). *Engaging with Climate Change: Psychoanalytic and Interdisciplinary Perspectives*. London: Routledge.

Zubala, A. and Karkou, V. (2015). Dance movement psychotherapy practice in the UK: Findings from the Arts Therapies Survey 2011. *Body, Movement and Dance in Psychotherapy: An International Journal for Theory, Research and Practice*, Vol. 10, No. 1, pp. 21–38.

Interruption 4

Dream

I am in the north London suburban garden of my childhood. The thick, green shrubs and trees that in reality line the boundary between one home and the next, now stand sparsely spaced, bare and with gaping holes that betray suburban privacy. The full moon lights the Earth in a clear, starry night. I catch sight of a burrow that I remember having dug the previous night – an underground labyrinth leading to a dark, secluded refuge, deep in the earth. My heart beats steadily within my ribcage that curves downwards from my horizontal spine. I sense the power in my shoulders and hips as four limbs propel me with intention along the boundary edge. I feel the gentle chill of the night beneath the thick fur that covers my skin, and I smell the musty richness and the pungent aromas of the soil.

An owl hoots. I pause a moment in the shadows, sniffing the air. My body tenses. There is a rustle in the bushes. I scuttle on my way, leaving small indentations in the uneven soil beneath me, and I stay close to the foliage that brushes against my fur. As I disappear into the darkness of the burrow, I wake with a start.

The room is lit by the full moon, the light radiating through the linen curtains. I sense my heart beating fast in my ribcage.

DOI: 10.4324/9781003322658-9

5 Ecopsychotherapy

An embodied immersion in environmental justice

The summer sun is mellowing. Golden leaves spiral downwards and shades of russet brown appear in rain-drenched bushes. The sun breaks through the clouds and silver-beaded raindrops slide slowly to the edge of leaves or hang suspended in spiders' webs.

I hear Maeve arriving. She knocks quietly, opening the door and peeping around the doorframe, asking,

'Is it OK to come in?'
'Of course!' I smile from my chair at the other end of the studio.

Maeve closes the door carefully, checking that it is shut. Looking down, she walks barefoot across the floor to join me. She pats the arms of the chair, looks at me and smiles, bringing her hands down to her lap. With a hint of a laugh, she says,

'Hello.'

She pauses. I am just taking a breath to greet her when she says,

'Is that how I should begin?'

Maeve looks around the room and then back at me. Her expression becomes serious.

'You know, I took the dog out this morning in the rain and it was so beautiful. Everything was dripping wet, the sun was shining and the smell of last night's rain was still fresh in the air.'

Maeve pauses. She looks down at either side of her feet, as if searching for something. She shifts position in her chair and her attention is caught

DOI: 10.4324/9781003322658-10

by something outside the window. I follow her gaze to see a tree blowing in the wind. Maeve looks back at me.

'I didn't even ask you how you were. Whatever must you think of me? So how are you?'

'I'm sitting here imagining you being out for a walk with your dog, feeling the sun on your skin and enjoying the smell of the rain.'

'Oh, it was so lovely. I really feel myself when I'm walking with the dog. You know, there's no one getting at you or criticising you or demanding something of you. Just me and the dog . . . and the world and the smell of the rain. Just walking and maybe finding blackberries or sweet chestnuts.'

Maeve pauses. I remember Maeve's previous disclosures of being criticised and put down by others.

'Actually,' she says,

'I was thinking, when I was out with the dog, about how it's so good to get away from all the talking.'

'Mm,' I say, wondering to myself if Maeve is indirectly asking for an invitation or prompt to guide her into movement.

'It's so easy to stay in the talking,' she says.

Maeve lifts her hands from her lap and begins to drum her fingers on the arms of the chair. She looks out into the studio space and then back at me, raising her eyebrows. Looking out into the space, she stretches her arms up to the ceiling.

'Perhaps you're thinking about getting away from the talking now and stepping into some movement,' I suggest.

'Yes, I think I will,' she says.

Maeve stands up and steps across the wooden floor to the centre of the studio. She turns to face me, puts her hands on her hips and her feet apart, standing in a patch of sunlight that is streaming through the window. I am struck by the uncharacteristic boldness of Maeve's position facing me and I also sense her discomfort. I wait, curbing my desire to rescue us both from the discomfort. I return her gaze, tilting my head to one side.

'How's that?' I ask.

'Er, actually, I don't like being here,' she says.

Maeve walks out of the patch of sunlight, to stand sideways, with the wall a few inches behind her.

'That's better,' she says.

Looking across the room at the wall opposite her, Maeve rolls her shoulders and twists from one side to the other, bending her elbows. She laces her fingers together and pushes the palms of her hands out in front of her and up above her head, lifting her shoulders and looking up. Maeve then opens her arms out to the side and downwards, to begin swinging them forwards and back by her hips, with a little bounce in her knees, still bouncing and swinging her arms playfully. She looks from one hand to the other and takes a step, shifting her weight backwards, forwards and side to side. Her upper body curves and stretches. In my mind's eye, I see her pulled by the current of the sea, as she moves fluidly with changes in direction and levels into the centre of the room and out again. I become completely absorbed in the directional flow of Maeve's movement. After some minutes, she pauses with her back to me and looks up, tilting her head with curiosity. She reaches both arms up towards one of the beams that runs across the room above her, rising onto her toes, as if trying to touch it. Maeve wobbles and puts her heels on the ground and her hands on her hips. She is now in the centre of the room.

The patch of sunlight has gone.

'It's like the barn we used to play in,' she says, looking along the beams, as if noticing them for the first time. Maeve drops her arms to her sides and turns to face me.

'I'll come and sit down,' she says, seeming suddenly self-conscious.

She quickly walks back to join me, and, sitting down, she brushes the fabric of her trousers with her hands and straightens her shirt. She glances quickly at me and then looks back up at the beams.

'Those beams are just like the ones in the barn at home where I used to play with my brothers and sisters. We'd make houses, we'd play hide and seek and we'd make swings on the beams.'

'Mmm,' I nod, looking up at the beams.

I imagine Maeve as a child, making a swing. I wonder out loud what Maeve remembered of that time.

'We were allowed to play in the barn and then in the field next to it. I loved being outside. The field sloped down to a stream and

I remember the water was always freezing, but we didn't care. We loved it; it was clear and fresh. I can feel that cold water on my skin now, just thinking about it. We had to get home before dark and we'd watch the sun drop slowly down behind the hill and then race back home before darkness fell. I remember a particular tree down by the river. I think it was an oak . . . a big, big tree with enormous branches and a wide trunk. When things got difficult at home, I would run down to the tree to feel safe. I told it all my troubles and it listened, particularly when my dad was angry.'

Ecological re-membering

Maeve had entered the session with her usual hesitation, almost as if she imagined that I wasn't expecting her. On reflecting this back in a later session, we explored Maeve's struggle to expect others to hold her in mind and her struggle to feel met in relationships. She arrived full of her morning walk, reflecting that she *really feels herself* when out walking the dog, and she contrasted this with her experience of unpredictable, volatile human relationships. I remembered previous disclosures she had made about flippant, derogatory micro-aggressions from her ex-partner and teenage children with regard to her looks, her ability and her accent, making her feel subordinated and reinforcing her sense of inadequacy. Maeve had also explored feeling overlooked and demeaned in relationships with the wider family, friends and colleagues. She compared herself unfavourably to her siblings' achievements in academia and business. She also recalled patterns of falling in love with men who, like her father, were mostly unavailable and at times abusive.

Maeve had grown up on a farm with her siblings, a volatile father and a loving mother, who was often unavailable due to excessive domestic demands. She remembered her father flying into a rage and lashing out in the noisy household that included several brothers, who also identified with the volatile male aggression. She remembered being told that she was useless and had internalised these powerful projections that sometimes manifest in the transference between her and me, as she might interpret my look as dismissive or contemptuous. She kept out of her father's way and learned that it was safer to be invisible. Yet, she also recalled the times when she experienced a softer, loving side of her father, most particularly when she joined him out in the fields to bring the cows in for milking. Maeve carried deep psychic, emotional wounds as a working-class woman and migrant, now reaching the menopause and fearing, as many women do, that she had missed any significant windows of life's opportunities. She yearned for personal and professional fulfilment as well as the permanency of a long-term, loving relationship.

As Maeve became immersed in the improvisational moving body in this session, she also got in touch with the embodied memories of her earth story.

The playful movement and the sight of the beams in the studio prompted memories of playing in the barn and out in the fields with her siblings. She recalled the cold-water stream, the sense of safety evoked by the powerful presence of the oak tree and her sense of well-being as she helped her father bring the cows in for milking. As Maeve recalled these memories, she was beginning to reconnect with an embodied, embedded subjectivity in which her sensing body remained alert, listening, responsive and playful as part of an intra-connected ecology of life. Maeve was exploring how her earth story manifests in her connection with the landscape, with the elements and with the other-than-human dance of the ecology.

This reconnection with an ecologically embedded identity is a vital component of the practice of ecopsychotherapy through which this chapter moves.

Ecopsychotherapy: an emergent field

Ecopsychotherapy has a rhizomatic heritage that has emerged from awareness and concern about the escalation of an environmentally destructive consumer culture in post-industrial capitalism that operates at the expense of the ecology. Rust (2020) notes that the term psych-ecology was used the 1960s (see Greenway, 1995), and the term ecopsychology was then coined by Roszak (1992) in his seminal text *The Voice of the Earth: An Exploration of Ecopsychology*. In this philosophical text, Roszak identified a direct connection between the mental health and well-being of humans and planetary health. These ideas were rumbling into existence amongst therapists, psychologists, environmental activists and social theorists in the Western world. Buzzell and Chalquist (2009) describe how ideas about ecopsychology were emerging within a small study group of scholars and activists in San Francisco in the early 1990s. Mental health and well-being needed to be reconceptualised in relation to wider discourses that included social, political and environmental justice. This thinking gave rise to the first anthology in the field entitled *Ecopsychology: Restoring the Earth, Healing the Mind* (Roszak et al., 1995). At around this time, therapists in the UK were also exploring the relationship between psychotherapy and anthropocentrism, posing questions about how individual internal worlds, socio-political organisational systems and the wider ecology of the earth's community are inextricably linked (Prentice, 2012, Rust, 2009). Since then, many anthologies representing the diverse nature of practices that have arisen (and are still arising) in this field have been published, for example, Buzzell and Chalquist (2009), Jordon and Hinds (2016), Rust and Totton (2012) and Weintrobe (2013), documenting some of the ways in which ecopsychology has developed into a wide range of well-being practices that embed human subjectivity in wider systemic webs of life. The field of ecopsychotherapy is an eclectic professional creature that continues to establish a professional identity (Dodds, 2013, Rust, 2020).

Emergent *eco* practices borrow from and synthesise philosophical and ethical ideas from deep ecology, outdoor practices and psychotherapeutic paradigms, along with critical theories that challenge individualistic values of advanced capitalism. Initially, the values, principles and practices struggled to gain visibility and recognition within mainstream services. In more recent years, with an increased conscious awareness about the climate emergency and environmental degradation and its impact on ecological communities, the interest in the imperative of ecopsychological theories, research and practices has expanded. Descriptors of these have included ecotherapy (Clinebell, 1996, Jordon & Hinds, 2016, Key & Tudor, 2023), ecopsychotherapy (Rust, 2020), wild therapy (Totton, 2011), equine psychotherapy (Hall, 2012), nature therapy (Berger & Tiry, 2012), environmental arts therapy (Siddons Heginworth, 2008) and horticultural therapy (Linden & Grut, 2002). What they all have in common is the premise that human subjectivity and ecological systems are mutually implicated. Fisher (2013) suggests that psychoanalysis itself was 'born only when the revolt of nature within the individual could no longer be ignored' (159). This came as the Western world was reaching a significant point of disconnection and increasing neurosis towards 'massive psychic derangement' (159) within an ideology of human exceptionalism, that is, the privileging of human desires over the needs of the wider ecological community and, indeed, over those humans who have not been included in that notion of humanhood fostered in the Enlightenment.

In a dream, I saw a young male client with schizophrenia standing on rocks on the island of Annet, a range of tall, jagged rocks rising from the surging Atlantic Sea. It is one of the most westerly Isles of the Scilly archipelago, 28 miles west of the coast of Cornwall, and is inhabited solely by birds. His foothold was unsteady, and he seemed resigned to being swept out to sea by a rolling wave. The deep ravines between the rocks and the inaccessibility of the island were sobering symbols, and, in the dream, I knew that he was struggling with serious mental illness. I wanted to reach him, but the terrain was too treacherous. This dream seemed to embody the idea of mental health as a symptom of the massive psychic derangement (Fisher, 2013) of a world that is edging into a dysfunctional system towards ecological collapse.

Ecological intra-subjectivity

Ecopsychotherapy invites discourses about intra-subjectivity that locate mental health in wider environmental, socio-cultural and political contexts, without diminishing the uniqueness of historical individual distress, as it manifests in mental health struggles. As Maeve's uniquely personal story unfolded within our therapeutic relationship, her story was held within a wider ecological web that included shifting identity politics. As we worked together, a rhizomatic assemblage emerged from the diffractive meeting places of unique individual experiences and powerful discourses of our time. Critical theories underpinning identity politics and social and environmental justice offered me a way of listening, a way of thinking and a way of challenging some of the biases that shaped my tendency to privilege some matters over others. For example, as Maeve began to remember her past, I listened attentively to the different kinds

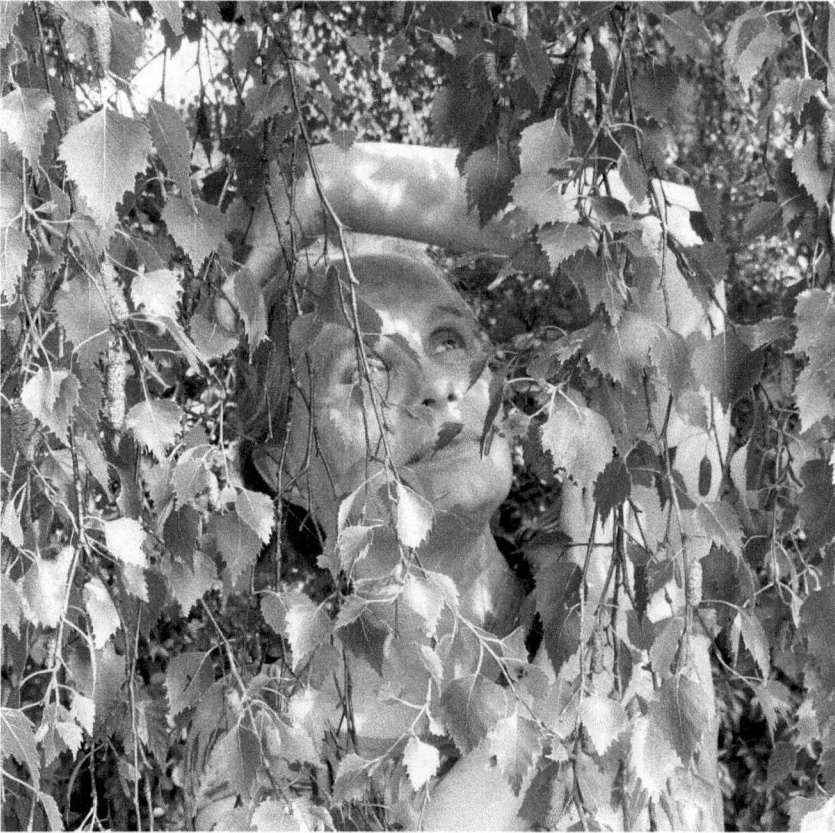

Figure 5.1 Re-membering.

of relationships that she described, human and more-than-human. I listened to what was being created in the immediate relationship between us, mapping out a rhizomatic assemblage of experiences as Maeve located herself within the material world through familial, social and environmental relationships.

She began re-membering her earth stories as she connected with an eco-logical selfhood. Maeve entered the session with the experience of walking her dog fresh in her mind that led her to an awareness of being in her moving body. As she was moving, she looked up at the beams in my studio, jogging her memory about the barn she used to play in as a child, and this memory led her to remember her connection to the land.

Ecological earth stories

Our earth stories are the deep and significant attachments that we make through, for example, our relationships with animals, building dens in the woods and finding refuge in the branches of a favourite tree. These are the special places, be it sand, rock, earth, water or grassland, that hold a particular significance in shaping who we have become and continue to become. At the end of this chapter, I offer you a provocation, and I wonder about the earth stories that will come to mind for you. Many clients express how they get in touch with their connection with the wider ecology in encounters with creatures, sand, sea, hills, mountains, lakes and other places that invite a material immersion in the human transversal entanglements within the ecology of a living earth. Listening for earth stories requires a commitment to the significance of attachments that move beyond the human realm. Barrows (1995) notes how in some cultures the birth of a child might be a time for rituals that honour the bonding between that newborn child and the earth, in which kinship expands beyond family 'to all living things and to the earth itself' (107). This conceptualises subjectivity as an intra-connected, ecological phenomenon, in which family, social and environmental ecologies are inseparable. This is how the *ecological self* is conceptualised.

Ecological selfhood

The term *ecological self* was coined by the Norwegian eco-philosopher and deep ecologist Naess (1995) and it provided a paradigm shift away from individualistic notions of human identity towards a conceptualisation of the self as a dynamic and intra-connected phenomenon. Naess (ibid) describes how, when involved in a scientific experiment, he saw a flea land in the middle of a drop of the chemical that he was investigating under a microscope. He watched in horror as the painful death of the flea was magnified before him, noting,

> If I had been *alienated* from the flea, not seeing intuitively anything even resembling myself, the death struggle would have left me feeling indifferent.
>
> (227)

Naess emphasises the significance of this empathic identification with the *other* that brings compassion and solidarity, deepening a realisation of the intra-connectedness of all life. The alternative is an alienation in which environmental destruction and degradation, like social and political injustices, become normalised as inevitable consequences of economic progress, productivity and profit. Economic growth comes at a cost and this alienation serves as an effective defence against feeling the grief in response to the devastating loss caused by environmental destruction.

Ecological selfhood invites a redefinition of the ways identities are organised and subjectivities conceived and performed. Ecological intra-dependence is the bedrock of ecopsychotherapy; hence, what we do to the earth, we do to ourselves and what we do to ourselves, we do to the earth. The idea of the ecological, intra-subjective-self shifts towards notions of selfhood that are implicated, entangled and located in the mutual dependency of a wider kinship.

Ecological loss and mourning

There are now many ecologically orientated therapists, activists and artists creating channels of expression to grieve and mourn environmental destruction and loss of biodiversity, as it is felt on a personal level. Buddhist scholar and environmental activist Joanna Macy (Macy & Young Brown, 1998) developed practice-based, facilitated programmes entitled The Work that Reconnects (ibid), providing a framework for identifying and expressing emotional responses to the ongoing losses of biodiversity. Without this capacity to process the grief, a pervasive process of denial (turning away) and disavowal (actively creating a narrative around the denial) can shut down thinking and feeling, obscuring the painful reality of the environmental destruction that is hard to face. Weintrobe (2013) identifies how disavowal operates at a less conscious level, actively distorting the truth of an unbearable reality. She explains how

> the more reality is systemically avoided through making it insignificant or through distortion, the more anxiety builds up unconsciously, and the greater the need to defend with further disavowal.
>
> (7)

We inhabit a socio-political system with an economic emphasis on growth that has become dependent on environmental destruction. The more we try to avoid our awareness of and complicity in this, the more we need to reinforce our denial and defend against it with disavowal. The violence of destruction within the system becomes normalised as we disconnect from an embodied, embedded empathic entanglement within an ecological web. Bernstein (2005) identifies a *borderland* phenomenon, referring to clients who are in touch with enormous despair in relation to the environmental destruction inherent in advanced capitalism. He describes a client who talks of carrying a 'Great Grief' (73) for the earth, describing it as an intimate part of himself. The highly specialised ego developed in the Western psyche, to which Bernstein refers, is fed by disavowal that allows us to hear alarming facts about environmental breakdown and continue with business as usual.

Some years ago, a friend gave me the beautiful book *The Lost Words* (Macfarlane & Morris, 2017) for my birthday. The book comprises poems dedicated to naming the trees, animals, plants and fruits that are disappearing from our vocabularies. These poems have also been set to music and provide an inspiration for improvisational movement that touches the heart of this climate crisis that we face. Species are rapidly disappearing. Gomes (2009) emphasises the significance of creating rituals to pay homage to these losses through 'alters of extinction' (246) that support an awakening and connection to the reality of environmental degradation. There are many things we can do as researchers and practitioners in acknowledging the *great grief* in which we are immersed, in our own lives and in that of our clients. In that grief, we can also find our love for each other and the world around us.

Ecological moving bodies

Maeve had an intuitive sense of the value of being *out with the dog* and of getting *away from all the talking*. As she moved into a place of embodied thinking, she found memories evoked that were sensory, playful, material connections with being in the world. Ecopsychotherapeutic practices will often bring clients back to the living breathing body to create a language that is responsive to the materiality of the world. For example, Kelvin Hall (2012), a psychotherapist who includes equine-assisted therapy in his practice, refers to a language of 'breath awareness, body position, gesture, timing, and more' (83). He describes a woman who wishes to connect to a horse, yet the subtle messages of domination in her body miss the 'invisible threads' (84) of the language of the wild herd and the horse shies away in alarm. Our embodied subjectivity is a potential place of connection, yet it is also infused with our cultural hegemony.

In a dream, I had been leaving one professional event and I was on my way to another. In the distance, on a nearby hill stood a family member who has been troubled all his life with serious mental illness. In that moment, I knew that if I acknowledged him, I would need to change my agenda and miss my scheduled event. I could pretend I hadn't seen him and carry on. I could just wave as I continued on my way. In the dream, I decided to approach him, knowing that in doing so I would compromise my plans. This dream stayed with me, and I remembered it whilst engaged in environmental movement on moorland. Crouching on the rock, I sensed the importance of the choices that I make, in turning to face the suffering, in allowing my compassion to underpin my decisions. As I gave the rock my full weight, feeling its solidity and breadth, I became acutely aware of how each choice that I make impacts the world and of the importance of turning to face the suffering, rather than passing it by with little more than a wave. We are all in this together, albeit differently and we are kinaesthetically connected through worlding processes (Bozalek & Fullager, 2022, Manning, 2012) that slow us down as we attend to the fabric of the world.

This concept of worlding is described by Manning (2012) as when

> the skin becomes not a container but a multidimensioned topological surface that folds in, through, and across spacetimes of experience, what emerges is not a self but the dynamic form of a worlding that refuses categorisation. Beyond the human, beyond their sense of touch or vision, beyond the object, what emerges is relation.
>
> (12)

This idea of worlding brings bodies into a relational material landscape that is the place of kinship.

Ecological adventures towards kinship

When 3-year-old Leila claimed 'I am the mountain' (Frizell, 2020: 211) in my community movement session, she was standing firm in her corporeal identity that recognised an ethically embodied, embedded identification with a wider material world. Relational moving bodies learn to be in the world and develop kinship through their intra-active, empathic participation and identification with differently moving bodies. Abram (2010) documents his learning from one of the medicine persons who he meets on his travels, describing how he finds a way to 'dream himself into the wild physicality of that Other' (ibid: 239) as he turns his attention to a raven. He finds his way into an empathic identification with the experience of the bird and, at the same time, finds he is reclaiming a part of himself. Abram's attunement to the raven enabled an expanded sense of his own becoming through the kinaesthetic, empathic experience that he describes.

In the book *Healing Fields* (Linden & Grut, 2002), psychotherapist Jenny Grut writes of her work at the Medical Foundation for the Care of Victims of Torture. These stories illustrate the power of using horticulture as a medium in psychotherapy for victims of torture, some of whom struggled with cultural and language differences and some of whom found therapy in enclosed rooms intolerable. Working on the land helped clients reconnect to memories of their homeland through digging in the earth, the cycles of growth and decay, the rain, sun and wind, which provided the materiality of experiences as touchstones to recall similarities and differences of their earth stories. Working outside on the land became an essential partner in reconfiguring shattered lives. In addition, Linden and Grut (ibid) note how 'stolen glimpses of vegetation through chinks of prison walls or barred windows' (19) provided political prisoners with small windows of hope in their despair. One client describes how he could see the top of a tree out of his prison window, and this became his connection with life itself. He had silent conversations with this tree that helped him maintain his connection with the world outside his cell. The changing seasons and the visiting birds kept him in touch with life itself, and he employed his imagination to create and maintain that connection.

I came across a beautiful poem published by the Koestler Trust,[1] in which a prisoner (Anonymous, 2017) describes a view from their cell window that is the long curve of the East Sussex Downs, which they liken to whales 'stranded on the unseen shore' (26). The second verse recalls a TV news item in which a family of whales are stranded, and the poet describes

whales, stranded like refugees,
Helpless victims of our tides,
With a one-way ticket to oblivion.
(ibid)

This poem brings together the grief of environmental degradation, in which whales become stranded and die on the shore, and the socio-political injustices of a growing refugee crisis, written by someone who, for whatever reason, has found themselves in prison and remains nameless in the publication of their poem. Who knows the story behind the creation of this poem and the decision to remain anonymous. It seems to me that *one-way ticket to oblivion* is an expression of existential grief for a world heading towards disaster, and we are all in this disaster together. No amount of status, power or wealth can save us, although it is the disadvantaged and the poor who suffer the impacts of this climate emergency disproportionately.

The return to our embodied earth stories offers a chance to move beyond the values of advanced capitalism that have contributed to the degradation of the earth and to find a way to reconnect to an ecological selfhood. At times, this work can be enhanced by stepping into the materiality of the landscape.

Ecological practising indoors and out

Historically, psychotherapy has taken place within the physical boundaries of a room. The emergence of ecopsychotherapy has brought with it the validation of outdoor therapy work, as different practices have been developed to foster empathic relationships within the ecology. As I look back on the dog-eared notebooks of my own personal therapy journal, I am reminded of the emancipatory power of a psychotherapy that (literally) followed the call of the woodpeckers into the shade of the ancient woodland, dogs sniffing around and racing out of sight, squirrels stopping to stare, wood anemones emerging from the shade as they spread their roots underground, butterflies dancing in the sun and spiders spinning fragile webs in the alcoves of trees, russet-brown leaves rocking gently to the ground and rooks' cries carrying eerily across the stark silhouettes of winter. My own therapy began in an indoor space, and after some discussion in response to my request as a client to go outside, a nearby ancient woodland became a regular context. The shifting seasons became an integral part of the diverse terrain of our encounter, amplifying the intra-active entanglement of client, therapist and environment in, and as, the fluctuating tides of the vitality of all matter.

After training as a DMP, I became increasingly interested in the emergent area of what I then knew as ecopsychology and ecotherapy. It was the turn of the century, the noughties, and ecopsychology presented a radical shift in anthropocentric ideas about selfhood, as well as offering a perspective on how DMP could be practised. I was developing my work as a DMP with learning-disabled children and young people who found it hard to respond to the traditional boundaries of therapy. I was treading lightly with what I could offer, with one eye on safe and ethical practice and another eye on what these children and young people needed and could tolerate. A theme that connected the stories of these children and young people and their families was the painful experience of not meeting the criteria for belonging. In the uncomfortable, thick fog of diversity, some of these families seemed to be clinging on to the edge of their communities, feeling like unwelcome wild plants in cultivated landscapes.

Primarily, my work was in schools for children and young people with complex needs, mostly in densely populated urban areas, and one of these schools happened to be situated on the edge of extensive parkland and woodland. The school was in an area of deprivation, and the pupils at the school were mainly from families who struggled financially. There was a tremendous sense of community in the local population, and there were also many mental health issues arising from social and economic deprivation and disadvantage. In addition, the families of these children and young people were struggling to manage life, with at least one member having complex needs, at a time when services were contracting.

I was working as a DMP with a group of six young teenagers aged between 12 and 14 years, supported by two teaching assistants. A few of these young people had never experienced any kind of holiday. Despite the extensive parkland and woodland next the school, they rarely had opportunities to play outside. Their able-bodied peers had begun to meet up with friends and explore the world together; however, these young teenagers were not equipped to manage in the world independently or, at least, without an accompanying adult. When they were not at school, they were usually confined to their homes, aside from some extra-curricular activities run by voluntary services. They mainly lived in high-rise flats, without gardens, and so had little access to outdoor areas. Journalist and author Louv (2005) warns of the dangers to children's mental health of restricted access to outdoor experiences, coining the term *nature-deficit disorder*, and these children had little access to environments other than the concrete of the city. The school would sometimes arrange activities in the nearby outdoor space, and together we discussed the possibility that some of the DMP work could take place outside. After careful thought, liaison with supporting staff and risk assessments, I took the idea to the young people that we could spend some of our therapy time out in the woods. *What did they think?* I asked. Grace, a teenager with Down's syndrome, was reading a cookery book.

'I know,' she said, commanding the attention of the group,
'Why don't we have pizza in the woods.'

Her book was opened on a page with a picture of oozing, melting cheese and bubbling tomato over a browned dough. This picture was safe, comforting and familiar for Grace, unlike my suggestion of going into the woods that perhaps seemed like a potentially unsafe and unfamiliar experience. Following Grace's lead, I asked the group how they might cook pizza in the woods, imagining that they might fantasise, as I was, about cooking in the open air. I imagined their connection to being kept warm and fed around the fire. Again, their thoughts were far from my imaginings. The consensus in the group was that we could call for a pizza delivery, which would arrive in a cardboard box via a man on a scooter.

With the support of the teaching assistants, we made a plan to visit the woods (without involving pizza) and, over the next few weeks, thought together about the idea. Finally, we made our first trip. Grace had been excited about the prospect of working outside; however, on arriving, she seemed disorientated. The group were playing grandmother's footsteps, intrigued by the added dimension of trying to walk quietly on the woodland floor of leaves and twigs. Grace removed herself from the immediate group, buried her head in her hands and sat on the ground by a tree with one of the teaching assistants sitting near her. Grace began to brush her hands along the ground, feeling the uneven textures on the woodland carpet. Her interest suddenly galvanised, she stood and moved a little further away from the group, drawn to a pile of fallen branches. She began to find twigs and branches from the surrounding area and carried them one by one to deposit them on the pile. Grace continued to heave increasingly heavy items onto her pile, making a den with the help of Nigel, the teaching assistant. When she finished, she welcomed the rest of the group over, describing to us the process of construction. All kinds of conversations ensued, for example, about creating spaces and establishing boundaries or about the plant, animal, bird and insect life around us. The young people responded to the kinaesthetic experience of this material environment and its inherent invitation of corporeal engagement. This making of a den in the woods was particularly significant for Grace, and she later referred to it repeatedly as a place that she called her *wood home* – a place of belonging and acceptance.

With Maeve, the work remained indoors; however, in working with the materiality of the space, with a sensitivity to the weather and the seasons, and in exploring her earth stories, often in movement improvisation and through the imagination, our work was grounded in ecological connection. With other clients, my practice at times is to begin indoors and, if outdoor work is to be a possibility, to think carefully together about what that might mean in terms of the therapeutic process, how we manage the boundaries of potentially being in a public place and how it might work practically. One of the places that I use for outdoor work is a tor on Dartmoor that is rarely frequented by walkers and visitors. It is high up and looks out over extensive views of moorland. For some clients, the exposure is overwhelming, and for others, it is inspirational. At times, glorious sunshine shifts to a deluge of rain in the space of one session, majestic rainbows appear and disappear, and sometimes clouds of fog descend. Ponies, sheep, birds and insects pass through the spot, as does the occasional human visitor, and we navigate this as and when it happens. We need to watch out for ticks at certain times of a year, and the exposed landscape requires different layers of clothes. Overall, the context is alive and sometimes unpredictable in a way that is different from an indoor space.

This outdoor work has presented interesting questions about how boundaries of safety are established and negotiated and challenges the notion that four walls and a closed door are essential elements of the therapeutic frame. Alaimo (2016) describes how we create the bounded spaces that we call homes that exist 'to keep outdoors, out-doors, defining the human as that which is protected within' (20). Taking therapy outside becomes a radical statement of ethical intent, a form of 'place-based activism' (ibid: 20) that locates the corporeal human subject within an embedded encounter with the landscape. What is crucial in working outside is that it is done with the deepest respect to

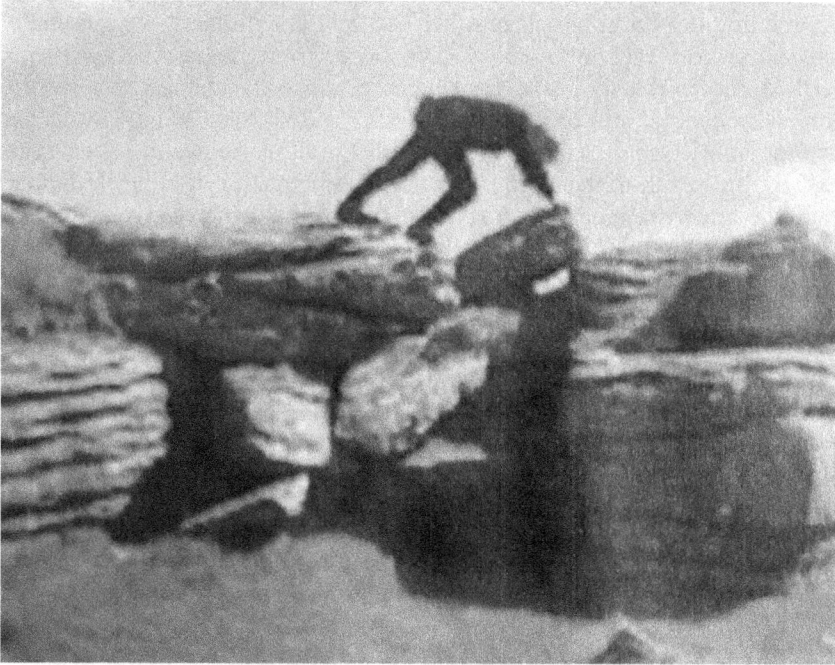

Figure 5.2 Ecological moving bodies.
Source: Photograph by the author.

landscape and the flora and fauna; otherwise, the natural world becomes, yet again, a resource to be consumed.

Ecologies in conclusions

In the same way that the emergence of psychotherapy over the last century has created a language to talk about psychic inner worlds and *inter*personal dynamics, so the emergent field of ecopsychotherapy is creating a language that embeds human *intra-subjectivity* in a wider systemic web of life – an *intrap*ersonal dynamic matrix within a material-discursive world. Ecopsychotherapy locates the identity of individual humans as implicitly implicated in the wider identity of the ecology. Knowledge comes from our experience of being *of* the world, rather than looking into the world from the outside. Being *of* the world is to be part of all matter, and all matter matters. There is a growing range of diverse practices within the field, underpinned by a conviction that mental health and well-being are enhanced as clients foster their connection as embodied, embedded creatures of this earth. In turn, a deeper connection to the natural material world around us fosters pro-environmental behaviour. There is not one way to practice. Ecological awareness can be fostered inside or out. It can be a lifeline to the prisoner who glimpses the landscape or a tree from their window. It can be, as Maeve noticed, a place of appreciation of how walk-ing the dog can bring her alive in her body. As practitioners, we can embed into our practice a way of listening and a way of prompting that brings clients' earth stories to the surface as part of the process of building resilience in a complicated world and of fostering empathy and kinship. As individuals and as a species, we are dependent on each other and on the health of the earth. In turn, the health of the earth is dependent on human behaviour. Individual identities are, therefore, embedded in this co-arising intricacy in which all be-ings are linked (Macey & Young, 1998).

Ecopsychotherapy is an anti-oppressive practice for environmental justice, and this cannot be separated from social and political justice. Concern about the environmental crisis has become increasingly evident on the mainstream stage, and at the same time, well-being practices with an ecological focus have become more commonplace in statutory and voluntary services. Within our advanced capitalist system, the focus on economic growth and the social, political and environmental decisions that support that growth have led to environmental degradation. We are all in this together; there is no outsider po-sition. In order to remain responsive to the impacts of environmental degrada-tion, it is necessary to get in touch with the grief and to mourn the enormous loss within the biodiversity of the planet. Haraway (2016) reminds us that

> (g)rief is a path to understanding entangled shared living and dying; human beings must grieve with, because we are in and of this fabric of undoing.
>
> (39)

One summer a few years ago, at the end of an ecopsychology outdoor tented conference, I was left with the beauty and power of the diversity of the life around me, with the damsel fly, dragonfly and butterfly darting through the net-tles, weaving their magic to welcome the midday summer sun. The goldfinches chasing from tree to tree called my attention to the mottled clouds that bil-lowed like silk and spread across the wide, open skies. The dance of the willows moved me, and my wonderment was brought to life by the kingfisher streaking along the meandering river in a flash of blue. The cool water in the river rippled gently and continuously downstream. The sand martins swooped in and out of their homes in the riverbank, twisting and turning high into the sky. A pigeon landed on top of the solar tent, holding a twig in her beak. She looked down at the ashes in the firepit from the previous night's community gathering. I re-membered the warm glow of the burning fire as darkness fell, and the figures that huddled around the burning logs shared their joy and their grief through poems, stories and music. This coming together creates chains of solidarity.

The notion of ecological selfhood is a place of entanglement that becomes unveiled as we connect to our earth stories, and these earth stories can bring us into an elemental kinship with the ecological dance of the material world that is already going on. As practitioners, it is essential that we turn our attention

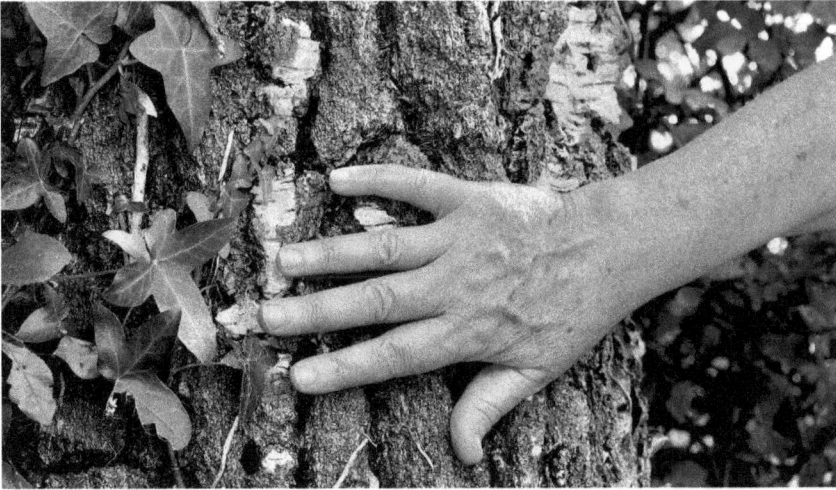

Figure 5.3 On touching the other.

Source: Photograph by the author.

to our own embodied sensitivity to the complex responsiveness of the ecology that is all around us. As Barad (2012) says,

> touching the Other is touching all Others, including the 'self', and touching the 'self' entails touching the strangers within.

(214)

Provocation

> You might like to spend a few moments, either alone or with a peer, reflecting on the landscapes that have been part of your life, in the city, the coast or countryside, mountains, lakes, trees, desert, city parks or suburban gardens; the wildlife that was significant and the domestic animals that shared your life.
>
> Using movement, art, music and/or creative writing, take yourself back into the landscapes that you have known. Remember the material, sensory memories in detail through your imagination, bringing back to life that part of your story that has shaped you.

Note

1 The Koestler Trust supports creativity in the arts, literature and science in the criminal justice system in the UK. See: https://koestlerarts.org.uk/about-us/the-history/

References

Abram, D. (2010). *Becoming Animal: An Earthly Cosmology*. New York: Pantheon Books.

Alaimo, S. (2016). *Exposed: Environmental Politics and Pleasures in Posthuman Times*. Minneapolis: University of Minnesota Press.

Anonymous. (2017). *Koestler Voices: New Poetry from Prisons, Vol. 1*. London: The Koestler Trust.

Barad, K. (2012). On touching – the inhuman that therefore I am. *Differences*, Vol. 23, No. 3, pp. 206–223.

Barrows, A. (1995). The ecopsychology of child development. In T. Roszak, M. Gomes and A. Kanner (eds.), *Ecopsychology: Restoring the Earth, Healing the Mind*, pp. 101–110. Los Angeles: Sierra Club Books.

Berger, R. and Tiry, M. (2012). The enchanting forest and the healing sand – nature therapy with people coping with psychiatric difficulties. *The Arts in Psychotherapy*, Vol. 39, No. 5, pp. 412–416.

Bernstein, J. (2005). *Living in the Borderland: The Evolution of Consciousness and the Challenge of Healing Trauma*. London: Routledge.

Bozalek, V. and Fullagar, S. (2022). Human/animal. In K. Murris (ed.), *A Glossary for Doing Postqualitative, New Materialist and Critical Posthumanist Research across Disciplines*, pp. 10–11. Oxon: Routledge.

Buzzell, L. and Chalquist, C. (2009). Psyche and nature in a circle of healing. In L. Buzzell and C. Chalquist (eds.), *Ecotherapy: Healing with Nature in Mind*, pp. 17–22. California, CA: Sierra Club Books.

Clinebell, H. (1996). *Ecotherapy; Healing Ourselves, Healing the Earth*. New York: Routledge.

Dodds, J. (2013). Minding the ecological body: Neuropsychoanalysis and ecopsychoanalysis. *Frontiers in Psychology*, Vol. 4, pp. 1–13.

Fisher, A. (2013). *Radical Ecopsychology: Psychology in the Service of Life*. New York: State University of New York Press.

Frizell, C. (2020). Reclaiming our innate vitality: Bringing embodied narratives to life through dance movement psychotherapy. In A. Williamson and B. Sellers-Young (eds.), *Spiritual Herstories: Call of the Soul in Dance Research*, pp. 207–220. Bristol: Intellect.

Gomes, M. (2009). Alters of extinction. In L. Buzzell and C. Chalquist (eds.), *Ecotherapy: Healing with Nature in Mind*, pp. 246–250. California, CA: Sierra Club Books.

Greenway, R. (1995). The wilderness effect and ecopsychology. In T. Roszak, A. Kanner and M. Gomes (eds.), *Ecopsychology: Restoring the Earth, Healing the Mind*, pp. 122–135. California, CA: Sierra Club Books.

Hall, K. (2012). Remembering the forgotten tongue. In M. J. Rust and N. Totton (eds.), *Vital Signs: Psychological Responses to Ecological Crisis*, pp. 79–88. London: Karnac.

Haraway, D. (2016). *Staying with the Trouble*. London: Duke University Press.

Jordon, M. and Hinds, J. (eds.). (2016). *Ecotherapy: Theory, Research and Practice*. London: Palgrave.

Key, D. and Tudor (2023). *Ecotherapy; A Field Guide*. London: Confer Ltd.

Linden, S. and Grut, J. (2002). *Healing Fields: Working with Psychotherapy and Nature to Rebuild Shattered Lives*. London: Frances Lincoln.

Louv, R. (2005). *Last Child in the Woods: Saving Our Children from Nature-Deficit Disorder*. New York: Algonquin Books.

Macfarlane, R. and Morris, J. (2017). *The Lost Words*. London: Penguin Books Ltd.

Macy, J. and Young Brown, M. (1998). *Coming Back to Life: Practices to Reconnect Our Lives: Our World*. Canada: New Society Publishers.

Manning, E. (2012). *Always More Than One: Individuation's Dance*. Durham: Duke University Press.

Naess, A. (1995). Self-realisation: An ecological approach to being in the world. In G. Sessions (ed.), *Deep Ecology for the 21st Century: Readings on the Philosophy and Practice of the New Environmentalism*, pp. 225–239. Boulder: Shambhala Publications.

Prentice, H. (2012). "Heart and soul": Inner and outer within the transition movement. In M. J. Rust and N. Totton (eds.), *Vital Signs: Psychological Responses to Ecological Crisis*, pp. 175–190. London: Karnac.

Roszak, T. (1992). *Voice of the Earth: An Exploration of Ecopsychology*. Grand Rapids: Phanes Press.

Roszak, T., Kanner, A. and Gomes, M. (eds.). (1995). *Ecopsychology: Restoring the Earth, Healing the Mind*. California, CA: Sierra Club Books.

Rust, M. J. (2009). Why and how do therapists become ecotherapists? In L. Buzzell and C. Chalquist (eds.), *Ecotherapy: Healing with Nature in Mind*, pp. 37–45. California, CA: Sierra Club Books.

Rust, M. J. (2020). *Towards an Ecopsychotherapy*. London: Confer Books.

Rust, M. J. and Totton, N. (eds.). (2012). *Vital Signs: Psychological Responses to Ecological Crisis*. London: Karnac.

Siddons Heginworth, I. (2008). *Environmental Arts Therapy and the Tree of Life*. Exeter: Spirits Rest Books.

Totton, N. (2011). *Wild Therapy*. Ross-on-Wye: PCCS Books.

Weintrobe, S. (ed.). (2013). *Engaging with Climate Change: Psychoanalytic and Interdisciplinary Perspectives*. London: Routledge.

Interruption 5

Coming down to earth[1]

Once I heard the story of a woman from the city who packed her bag and headed north. Arriving at a coastal wilderness, she wandered across the beach in search of purpose, balancing on boulders and peering inquisitively through giant stepping stones. Smaller rocks lay on still smaller stones that harboured glistening pebbles and spiralling shells. She trod lightly, catching her balance at every step and breathing with the roar of rushing waves that brushed against tendrils of clinging sea anemones as push dissolved into pull. The woman inhaled vibrant sea air that rushed through her veins, tossing her imagination like flotsam across the shoreline into the open sea and back onto the beach. She edged her way towards the waves, in search of reason.

'What is your intention?' the woman cried into a wave that lapped gently towards her before softly caressing the sand on its retreat.
'We have no use for intention,' it whispered.
'We dance with the rhythms of Earth and follow the wisdom of Moon. We rise and fall with the spirits of Ocean and flow with currents of Time.'

The next morning, the woman rose before dawn and headed along the coast, intending to find a place to settle until dusk. She took a flask of water, clothes to keep her warm and a torch to guide her home. The sun rose and she climbed a rock, pausing momentarily to watch a seal swimming in a bay. Continuing to climb, she found a small plateau overlooking jagged rocks that rose ominously from rounded boulders below. The sea lurched against the rocks, engulfing them in green-grey water with a thundering roar, before retreating to expose the glistening stone. Chill sea air brushed against her cheek and she caught sight of silver ripples in the wake of a sea otter flipping effortlessly from one side to the other and she pushed through the water. The rhythmic swell of gently billowing silver waves was reaching, pulling, filling and emptying. Light rain began to fall, landing like crystal balls on the surface tension in rock pools below. The rain stopped and the water in the rock pools smoothed into mirrors, reflecting scudding clouds. The woman surrendered to the urge to sleep and curled into a nearby rock, which fitted around her like a glove. Her hip nestled into a concave space and her legs curled around its base. Her elbow and shoulder found

DOI: 10.4324/9781003322658-11

a comfortable niche and a pillow of stone supported her head. Rain was falling again. The woman closed her eyes and was rocked to sleep by a lullaby of rushing waves, crying gulls and the continuous pattering of rain on the hood of her raincoat. She felt herself sinking to the centre of the earth. Time moved around as the earth slowly shifted its relationship to the sun, which lit the world from behind a veil of clouds. The rain continued. Waves crashed against the rocks. Gulls screeched overhead. The voluminous sea closed in over the rock pools and the sun began its descent towards the horizon.

The woman began to stir, conscious of a rumbling from the rock beneath her. The rock became her ribs, wrapping around her heart and gently breathing through her. She became the rhythm of the rock and the heartbeat of the earth, suspended in the liminality of a waking dreamtime. She drifted into a vision of death dissolving her flesh – bare bones lying upon the rock to be washed into the sea by a giant wave, before sinking down into the fathomless depths of the ocean to begin a slow transformation into the rocks on which future women will sleep.

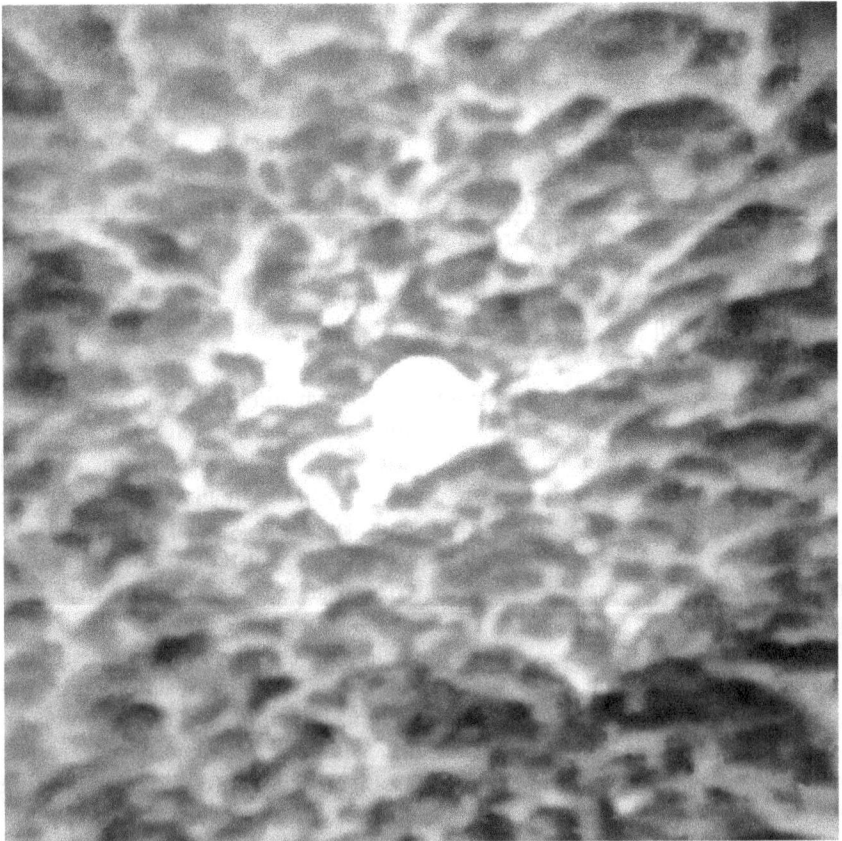

Figure 5a.1 Harvest moon rising behind mottled clouds.
Source: Photograph by the author.

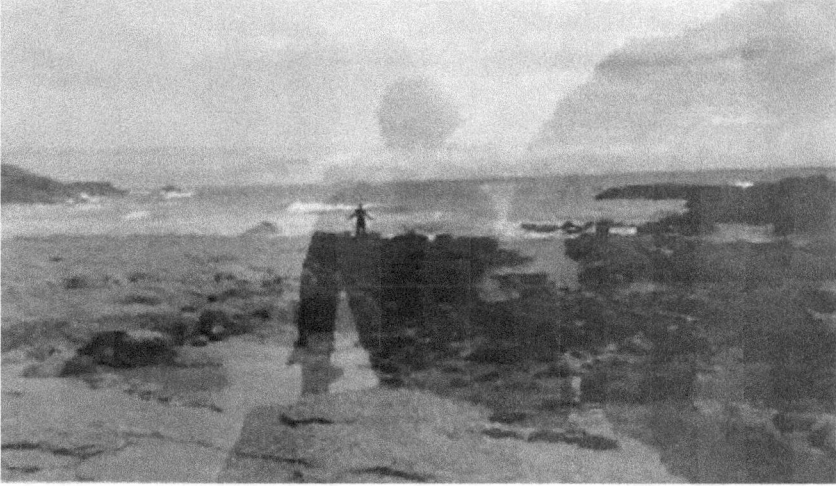

Figure 5a.2 Rocks and sea.

Source: Photograph by Alan Armitage.

The rain stopped and a break in the clouds freed a shaft of sunlight from the sky, throwing a silver pathway towards the distant horizon. Gannets plunged head first into the sea. Cormorants skimmed the surface of the ocean and oyster catchers tore across the bay with whooping cries and fast beating wings.

The light was dimming. A harvest moon was rising behind mottled clouds.

The woman gathered her belongings and headed back by the light of her torch to re-enter the human realm with caution.

The next morning, she rose before dawn and made her way up a muddy hill, sodden from the rain. She turned and stood high above the shoreline, watching as the earth shifted towards the dawn, transforming the silhouettes of the landscape into rich autumn colours in the yellow-orange hue of the gathering morning light. Stags whispered from the shadows. With the deep red mountains behind her, she stood on the top of the world, gazing into the visceral body of the universe.

She listened for the silence beneath the urgent sound of rushing waves.

The woman returned to the city to stand on a crowded tube train, strangely unperturbed by the shoulder-to-shoulder bustle of city life. Closing her eyes, she remembered the living, breathing earth beneath the morning rush hour.

Note

1 This story is adapted from the original publication in: Frizell (2008).

Reference

Frizell, C. (2008). Coming down to earth. e-motion , Vol. XVIII, No. 1. 1460–1281, pp. 8–10.

6 Research as practice

Practice-led inquiry

'Here is a printed copy of the information sheet I sent you.'

I lift the papers on my lap about an inch into the air, clasping them between the thumb and index finger of each hand.

'. . . and I was wondering if you had any thoughts . . . or comments . . . or questions.'

I replace the papers on my lap silently, hearing the formal tone of my voice and balking at my stumbling words. Maeve tilts her head expectantly and raises her eyebrows. I separate her copy and hand it to her and she smiles with an aliveness in her gaze. Looking at the paper, she rests her wrists on her knees. I sit back into my chair, crossing one leg over the other, holding my information sheet awkwardly in front of me. Maeve looks alternately between the information sheet and me.

'Yes, I did read it,' she says.

She taps the toes of both feet rhythmically on the carpet. Falling leaves swirl past the widow in a strong gust of wind. The air in the room is still. I hear the clock ticking. Maeve looks at her sheet, tilting her head from side to side. She takes a deliberate breath in and rocks back in her chair. Stretching her legs along the floor, she looks at me, saying,

'I suppose . . . I'm nervous of what might come out.'

She runs her bottom lip across her top teeth.

'I don't know what I might say . . . what you might write about. And when I read the . . .. '

DOI: 10.4324/9781003322658-12

She frowns and checks the heading at the top of the page,

'The in-for-ma-tion sheet.'

I am not sure if she has finished. I nod, taking air in through my nostrils and I look back at the heading *information sheet*, surprised to find that in this moment, I have a kind of contempt towards it. I look back at Maeve, who is looking at me, expectantly, perhaps provocatively.
   I consciously take another breath.

'When you read the information sheet?' I ask.

Maeve looks at more leaves swirling past the window in another gust of wind.

'I suppose what I'm saying is that I feel a mixture of excitement and I'm also nervous. But that's probably as much about coming here as anything.'

Maeve's concerns land in my body, like a single leaf suspended in its downward spiral. I struggle with an urge to reassure her; *I have done my homework; it will all work out well*, I want to say, but instead respond with,

'That's understandable. There's no pressure to participate and even if you agree to, you can withdraw from the project at any time . . . up to the date stated on the form. You can take your time to decide either way.'

As I speak these words, I am aware that they are falling short of the complexity of this thing through which we are struggling. I run my index finger across the indented heading that articulates this reminder. My foot twitches as I struggle with my neutrality.

'Yes,' she says, looking at her copy.
   'I mean . . . what if there are things that I don't want to have recorded? What then?'
   'Yes, of course. There might be things that you don't want to be included in the research. That can be in your hands. At the end, I will send you the information that I would like to use and you can agree to it or not. And any information would be anonymous, you know . . . changing your name . . . and any details that might identify you.'

> Maeve nods. Something settles inside me.
>
> 'I also wonder if *you're* wondering if you can trust me.'
>
> Maeve's face becomes serious. She looks down.

Research contracting

Maeve initially contacted me in response to a call for research participants for a case-study inquiry that proposed a DMP intervention of 40 weekly sessions with individual clients. The inquiry set out to interrogate the processes of individual DMP through a psychodynamic, ecofeminist lens, exploring the therapeutic process as it manifests within an intra-active, rhizomatic assemblage. The focus of the inquiry was on my experience as a practitioner within the entanglement of the relationship. In the vignette above, Maeve and I were moving into the ethical landscape of what it might mean to participate in a therapeutic relationship as research fieldwork. Maeve was articulating the vulnerability that runs through the fabric of research and practice in her questions about what might be revealed and how I might use the data. In addition, I picked up on less conscious power differentials (perceived and actual) diffracting between us, as a potential therapist and client and as a potential researcher and research participant. This exchange might be read from many vertices that are diffracting simultaneously and at the end of the vignette above, I wondered out loud if one of these vertices was that of trust, as a fluctuating, dynamic process, rather than a one-off event. Trust moved through the ebbs and flows of the transference and countertransference dynamics that constellated between us. On the surface, it was a practical arrangement between two people about a decision to engage in a research project or not and this was entangled with a potential formation of a therapeutic alliance, with all the less conscious phenomena intra-acting in that field, including the corporeal power differentials at play.

As a researcher, I was just one part of a greater assemblage and not the most important (Lather, 2013). I found myself muddling through my complex role as a practitioner-researcher and researcher-practitioner. The reality of the processes in action (as always) was more complex than the theory. At this point of meeting Maeve to discuss her participation, I had written a research proposal and secured ethical approval at Goldsmiths, University of London, where I work, designing a project and creating an information sheet and consent form. These formal processes then became entangled within the emergent relational processes of recruitment for the research fieldwork. The information sheet and consent form became material actors in this dance and I was surprised to find a fleeting feeling of contempt towards the information sheet. When I explored this more fully in supervision, I realised that it had become a powerful actor in a complex relational process, representing an authority that held its own story of oppressive academic discourses that were entangled with my own history.

Maeve had had previous experience of verbal psychotherapy and was drawn to this research partly through curiosity based on her prior experience, partly by her fascination in working with the creative moving body through DMP and partly by the idea of 40 sessions free of charge. I sensed Maeve's am-bivalence and I did not want to rush her into taking a decision either way. In my own supervision, I explored that tension between my own less conscious desire for Maeve to participate and my capacity to facilitate a well-informed decision. Neutrality as an ethical principle became bound into my inevitable active participation in the relational process.

This is an example of the ethical dimensions of recruiting participants for practice-led research projects – both the formal ethical processes and the more subtle embodied ethics at play at less conscious levels. The procedure of fi-nalising the paperwork creates a sense that something is being formed and an illusion of order, unlike the hands-on, relational process of the experience of working together in the room. The ethics of consent comprises multi-layered, sometimes messy, dialogic processes that take place as an improvisation over time, rather than as a scripted event.

Research as ethical landscapes

Ethics applications are scrutinised and approved through formal processes that give the green light for research fieldwork. This formality requires the researcher to conceptualise the project as a whole and to demonstrate risk assessments that anticipate and address potential conflicts. The researcher needs to demonstrate how potential participants will be given every oppor-tunity to make an informed choice about their decision. The process is a useful reflective space about respecting the participative agency and integrity of potential participants, with a focus on working in their best interests. It demands a thoughtfulness about the power differentials that might poten-tially adversely impact respective participants' experiences. Being granted ethical approval is a springboard to begin recruitment, with a commitment to creating ethico-onto-epistemological[1] assemblages that are ongoing.

There are many layers to the ethics of research recruitment and each time I engage with this process, it is different. For example, in recruiting children and teenagers as research participants, formal consent is officially gained from parents; however, there is also an ethical imperative to gain consent from the children and young people themselves. A further complexity might be if these children and young people are, for example, learning-disabled and/or for whom verbal language and cognitive understanding is not their preferred or useful form of communication. This then presents a dilemma for the re-searcher, as it does also for gaining consent for therapeutic practice, presenting the question of how we demonstrate professional accountability for issues of consent. Those working in the arts therapies develop skills to maintain a sensitivity and alertness to working with consent as a process over time, which does not necessarily involve language as the primary channel. Consent for both research and practice emerges through relational interplay and the arts provide alternative ways of mediating consent as an intra-active, more-than-verbal process over time, rather than as a finite event. It is important that the exploration of consent is not rushed. It is also crucial that consent is a continuous negotiation that moves beyond the initial mutual agreement to begin the work.

I remember recruiting participants for a DMP case-study research project with learning-disabled children. Julie had been referred as a potential participant and I first visited her in her classroom. I had already held an information session for school staff and another for parents of potential participants. Julie's mother had consented enthusiastically to the possibility of Julie's participation. I needed to spend some time introducing myself to Julie, ascertaining how I might present the idea of working together in a practice-led research project and request her consent. I had some ideas, as well as some resources, such as visual representants and prompts to support an explanation of the process that I had used previously; however, firstly, I needed to get a sense of what constellated relationally between Julie and me. This initial intra-action can be found in *Interruption 1: Have you come to see her?* (pages 21–22). In this initial encounter with Julie, I was struck by her relationship with spoken language that was textural, rhythmic and with its own logic that I took time to understand. I was intrigued by her rhythmic play with my name and then sentences repeated with a change of emphasis. Julie had shown little interest in the classroom task and after my brief initial meeting with her, I was left with feelings of emptiness. I found my mind wandering to the other children in the class and I noticed how hard it was to keep Julie in mind. The following week, as had been agreed with Julie's mother and the staff, Julie came along to my therapy room in the school for an initial assessment for the research project. She was immediately drawn to the puppets in the room, and these became central players in thinking through the idea of working together. Another resource that became key to our process together was a mirror. Julie was captivated by her own image and I had a greater sense of our relationship when we worked through the mirror. We worked with the idea of consent, both implicit and explicit, and this was a process over several sessions. Consent as a phenomenon was partially an implicit idea, for example, in Julie's willingness to return to the therapy room the following week and I was careful to avoid any kind of even subtle coercion from any of the adults around her. Explicitly, we worked with the puppets, as externalising the ideas seemed a safer place for Julie. We also played with Julie's reflection in the mirror, particularly through sound and rhythm. Julie gradually began to understand that she was an active agent in our relationship. In an early meeting with Julie's mother, I learned that just before Julie was born, a key member of the family had committed suicide and so Julie had entered the world in an atmosphere of grief and despair. Those charged with her care had little emotional space available for her. I realised that my difficulty in holding her in mind and my drowsiness that manifest in sessions were most likely a powerful projective identification. Although Julie's mother had willingly signed the consent form, what was more difficult to glean was Julie's understanding of what it meant to be a research participant. This is a dilemma for researchers recruiting participants for whom language and cognition are not prominent modes of experience, and the Mental Capacity Act[2] offers important guidelines to support researchers' thinking around this. Doubts about the capacity to consent, along with power differentials that may result in learning-disabled people being more susceptible to coercion, might deter research in this area. However, excluding learning-disabled people as potential participants on this basis might itself constitute discrimination (Goldsmith & Skirton, 2015). Researching that leads to publications can give an important voice and visibility to the work that researching-practitioners do with people who live at the margins and for whom it is important to develop and share innovative practice. It is also important that, as researchers and practitioners, we use our professional privilege ethically and responsibly, with humility and always in participants' best interests. I wonder how you, as the reader, position yourself in relation to this dilemma.

Research trajectories from qualitative to postqualitative

Before considering myself a researcher, I had a vague notion of research as alienating and exclusive. For many years, I was not in a financial or practical position to embark on PhD. I also imagined that engaging in research would take me away from the practice as a community dance artist, a DMP and a higher education institution educator that I found fulfilling. Perhaps less consciously, I was waiting for someone to invite me into a research world that I perceived as elitist and *other*. My experience of working at a university, however, was to find myself surrounded by inspiring researchers committed to creative processes that engaged with the subtleties of human relationships and moved within the contradictions of different ways of knowledge-ing the world. I realised that research could be playful and practice-led and this realisation challenged a powerful and pervasive myth that I had internalised with regard to the exceptionalism and elitism of research. I was given opportunities to learn by assisting researcher-colleagues in their projects, working alongside them and realising the importance and significance of critical inquiry in the field of professional practice.

I then began to embark on leading my own research projects, beginning with qualitative research, for example, using practice-led, qualitative inquiry into the 'production of *reflexive knowing*' (McLeod, 2001: 3), exploring the process of group supervision (Frizell, 2012). I presented the findings in a peer-reviewed article, illustrating how creative moving bodies in the process of active imagination enabled supervisees to access less-conscious processes impacting on attitudes towards learning disability. Reflexivity was central to my thinking at this time and as I later began to immerse myself in posthuman and new materialist ecofeminist thinking, I found the concept of reflexivity to be problematised as a phenomenon that can simply reinforce the existing subjectivity of the therapist, returning to what we already think that we know.

Linnell (2006) suggests that

> (a)t the limits of reflexivity I do not so much turn as become the turn itself, that which is always forming through turning towards the Other, losing myself at the moment of self-consciousness, finding myself only in that which I must strive to, but cannot, know.
>
> (105)

This distinction between turning and becoming the turn is the place of indeterminacy and vulnerability that intra-acts within the very thing that is trying to be thought about. As we sink into a place of reflexivity, we are in danger of returning to the comfort of reinforcing and reproducing what we already knew, rather than allowing ourselves to return within an intra-active, emergent world into a place of immanence.

I moved through practice-led research methods, responding to opportunities to join communities of authors in collected anthologies. These included exploring DMP with learning-disabled clients (Unkovich et al., 2017), exploring links between the environmental crisis and mental health and how these issues underpinned new discourses in psychotherapy (Frizell, 2014) and joining 21 women authors from a wide range of somatic movement and dance studies, offering interdisciplinary, practice-led research methods that challenged cultural hegemonies (Williamson & Sellers-Young, 2020). At the same time, I was taking a sideways step into interpretive phenomenological analysis (IPA) (Smith et al., 2012), a methodological framework that supported semi-structured focus groups and interviews. One of these projects, co-facilitated with an inspirational researcher-colleague, David Woodger,[3] comprised in-depth focus groups and interviews with some of the most complex and vulnerable children and young people in the UK who had a history of being excluded from school (Frizell & Woodger, 2019).

I realised that this evolving body of practice-led research was problematising notions of selfhood and subjectivity, referencing inclusion, normalcy and kinship and I was increasingly drawing on new materialism and posthumanism. A particular event in the process of the research served as a provocation to think differently about research methodology. It might be considered an example of *data that glow*, that is, when small fragments of the research material intensify our gaze and make us pause 'to burrow inside it' (MacLure, 2010: 282) for no logical reason. MacLure (2010) describes the process of discovering *data that glow* as when

> some detail . . . starts to glimmer, gathering our attention. Things both slow down and speed up.
>
> (ibid: 282)

And data unexpectedly reveal themselves to us. I was using IPA as a method to conduct interviews with parents, asking about their experience of discovering the news that their child had Down's syndrome. The night before visiting one mother, I dreamt about a newborn foal who attracted onlookers' curiosity by virtue of being different. In the interview the next day, the mother mentioned that her older daughter had wondered about horses being born with Down's syndrome. At this point in the interview, the cat jumped onto the table, knocking the recording equipment on the floor and nuzzling her head against me, making it hard to continue. This moment appeared in the transcription as a clatter, yet my mind kept returning to the synchronicity of the dream, the mother's account of her daughter's reflections on horses and the cat's interruption. This sequence of events proved a pivotal line of flight in shifting my thinking about what it means to be human, as well as some of the humanist assumptions that we might be making in research practice (Frizell, 2023). I was arriving into postqualitative inquiry.

Research as postqualitative inquiry

As I developed as a qualitative researcher, I encountered methodological challenges and limitations. I was drawn to the idea that if methodology is separated from epistemology and ontology, it is in danger of becoming formulaic, with a tendency towards mechanised techniques (St Pierre, 2014). Lather (2013) asserts that new ways of thinking can materialise as we shift from binary thinking (i.e., defining this from that) into multiplicities (i.e., holding different and sometimes contradictory possibilities simultaneously), staying with material-discursive tensions and contradictions that problematise the process. The ways in which the human subject has been conceptualised in Western thought are underpinned by a metaphysical and scientific 'colonising binary logic' (Murris, 2021: 68), and postqualitative inquiry disrupts assumptions that support this logic. In order to generate new knowledge about the world, as researchers, we need to problematise methodological inquiry by questioning the way we are thinking about the existence of that world, the ways in which we are understanding that world through knowledge and what it is that we consider constitutes knowledge.

In order to discover new ways of thinking, I began to take my place within the ebbs and flows of intra-acting research assemblages, remaining 'responsible and responsive to the world's patternings and murmurings' (Barad, 2012: 207). Barad (2007) challenges interiority and exteriority as binaries, suggesting that they are not determined, inseparable phenomena. Rather, she posits notions of 'exteriority within' (177) that locates all phenomena (including the researcher) within entangled webs of matter and discourse. The researcher's gaze, then, is intricately entangled with the subject (rather than object) of that gaze, situating 'all bodies, human and nonhuman, in relations of matter and mattering' (MacDonald & Wiens, 2019: 366). In the vignette that opens this chapter, I struggled with the tension between the principle of neutrality and

my situatedness within a process, concluding that what is valuable is the struggle itself. In this web of intra-connectedness, it is the processual relations of
difference that are important, within emergent diffractive patterns, rather than
the notion of phenomena as pre-existing entities.

Research through rhizomatic assemblages

An ecofeminist approach, arising from new materialist and posthumanist
ethico-onto-epistemologies, welcomes the agency of more-than-human and
material collaborators, organic, non-organic and technological within the
affective capacity of things.[4] Rhizomatic constellations invite the non-linear
emergence of phenomena across spatial, temporal and material landscapes
(*spacetimemattering*) and hold contradictions and multiplicities, welcoming
interruptions as lines of flight that can open pathways into new insights. Concepts such as rhizomatic assemblages and diffractive analysis have enabled me,
as a researcher, to create a container for the fluidity and complexity of ecofeminist values.

The idea of a research assemblage is a relational gathering of material-
discursive matters. Assemblages are dynamic and processual by nature, bringing a focus to relational potential, that is, 'of becoming rather than being'
(Deleuze & Guattari, 1987: 275). Within assemblages, there are stabilising
flows of territorialisation and de-territorialising flows that are de-stabilising,
leading to constituent lines of flight (Deleuze & Guattari, 1987). The component parts of the assemblage bump up against each other, affecting each other
from within, creating an always-in-process production of knowledge that
employs an 'affect economy' (Fox & Alldred, 2015: 405), with an orientation
towards

> processes and flows rather than structures and stable forms; to matters
> of power and resistance; and to interactions that draw small and large
> relations into assemblage.
>
> (ibid: 407)

The dynamic, relational processes within assemblages are characterised by
permeability, plurality and multiplicity with blurred, rather than definitive,
boundaries between phenomena. Bennett (2010) describes assemblages as

> living, throbbing confederations that are able to function despite the
> persistent presence of energies that confound them from within.
>
> (ibid: 23)

An example of the emergence of a research assemblage was my project *Cliff Moves*.
This inquiry brought together ideas about the experience and performance of improvisational moving bodies in relation to ecofeminist, posthuman principles. As
a research project, it was in an emergent and embryonic stage just after the winter

solstice of 2019. With the intention of having a break, a spontaneous instinct took me to the tin mines at Botallack, on the west coast of Cornwall. I followed the rugged coast from Zennor to St Ives (see *Prologue: Cliff moves*, pages 1–2) and, on arriving at St Ives, came across an exhibition entitled 'From where I stand' (Nkanga, 2019) by performance artist Otobong Nkanga at the Tate St Ives gallery. As I wandered through the exhibition in muddy walking boots, I realised that this exhibition clearly resonated thematically with my research ideas. In my attempt to take a break from this research, I had, in fact, walked (literally) further into it! The glow of its significance did not fade, and I began to conceptualise a repeat of this walk as participatory-performance-as-research. Although convinced of the significance of this experience, what was less clear was the *how* in terms of giving such data a voice in this process of immanence. As the planning was underway, the pandemic struck, interrupting my intentions of creating a performance. I then realised that a performance of some kind had, unknowingly to me, already revealed itself, within a synchronous time inversion. Data were glowing from unexpected places, and a potential performance seemed to be welcoming '(t)he "disorderliness" of the creative process' (Trimingham, 2002: 56) into the inquiry.

The prospect of a wild walk performance continued to tap on the window of my attention. Glancing through the glass pane of my imagination, I saw a long-eared animal racing across the field towards the horizon, silhouetted against the late afternoon moon.

A hare!

Of course!

A creature of the moon and the night. The symbol of fertility and creativity.

A shapeshifter.

A hare-brained[5] idea was calling to be born, bringing together bodies that were creating a narrative, 'affecting one another and generating intensities' (Stewart, 2007: 128): breathing bodies, bodies without lungs, bodies of discourse, bodies of thinking, elemental bodies and bodies without organs (Deluze & Guattari, 1987: 150).[6] All players within this assemblage were affecting and being affected by each other in a rhizomatic configuration, bringing forth a form of knowledge-ing grounded in what it was doing, rather than the meaning it was creating (LaMothe, 2015, Markula, 2006).

Researching through the agency of the camera (for example)

My intention of a live performance became disrupted by the uncertainty of how the COVID-19 pandemic would unfold. Perhaps a film of some kind might be feasible in developing the theme of the research. Unsure that restrictions would allow me to revisit the walk, I began to explore the idea of filming movement, within the reality of social and geographical restrictions.

But if I was going to make a film, then I would need a camera.

I ordered a camcorder and tripod online. The doorbell rang. The equipment arrived. Charging the battery took time. Once charged, I set up the camera. It looked back at me, and the screen said *insert memory card*. Naively, I had not realised that I needed to purchase this separately. I ordered the memory card and, before it arrived, watched the camera standing on its tripod without a memory, looking back at me with its unseeing lens. I reflected on its potential to allow 'the private to become public' (Skaife et al., 2020: 56) and noticed a sense of excitement combined with nervousness.

The objectifying lens of the camera might be considered nothing more than a technical apparatus; however, already it was bringing an agency of its own. I glanced at the still unseeing lens of my newly acquired camera, wondering how its memory, currently ex situ, would disrupt this research. I attached the camera to a tripod, angling the lens and stepping into the frame, like Alice into the looking glass. The camera stood on its tripod, and I became familiar with its statuesque form. The memory card arrived. I installed it and entered the garden with camera and tripod to become newly entangled in the world's performance. When I eventually began to film on a local beach, I moved tentatively towards the eye of the camera, as if towards a cliff edge.

I stepped into the cinematic frame and glanced at the lens looking back at me, wondering how it would remember these improvised scores performed in a 'deeply site-sensitive, time-sensitive, and person-sensitive process' (Ashley,

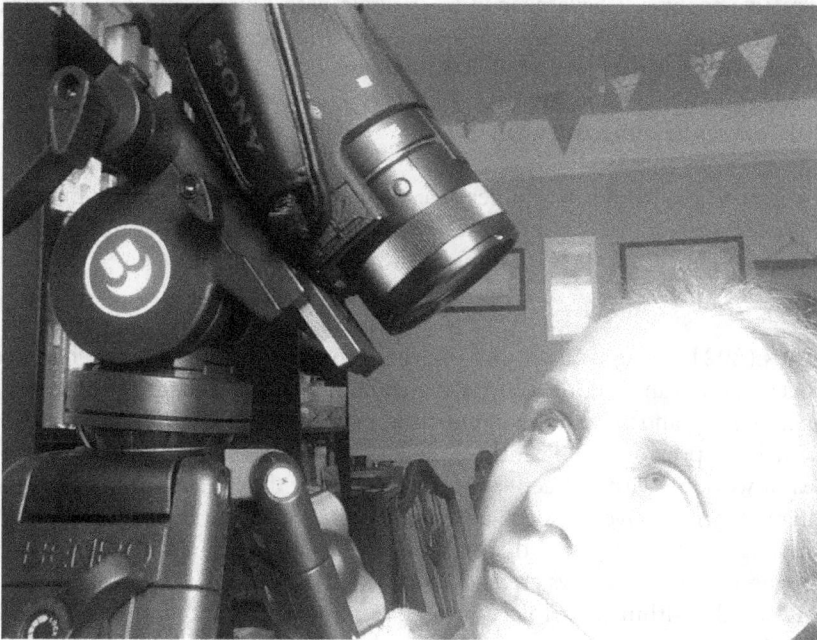

Figure 6.1 Camera.
Source: Selfie by the author.

2019: 595) connecting me to this place through 'specific microrelations' (ibid) in which I was entangled. I moved amongst iterative processes that enable me to open a space for practice-led knowledge-ing to be generated. I considered that these images memorised by the camera were 'very explicitly made, not taken' (Reason, 2012: 239).

This is an example of the interdisciplinary and transdisciplinary potential of creating research assemblages that invite diffractive processes across discourse(s) and matter(s), investigating 'patterns of interference' (Davies, 2014: 740) within encounters, finding flows of differences and reading and moving data through each other, noticing the diffractions that occur (Lenz Taguchi & Palmer, 2013). It is a slow process.

Research through diffractive analysis

Barad (2007, 2014) describes diffractive methodology as a process of

> reading insights through one another in attending and responding to the details and specificities of relations of difference and how they matter.
>
> (Barad, 2007: 71)

Diffraction is about convergence, divergence and the multiple possibilities of becoming that are created in the collision of things, that is, a 'cutting together-apart' (Barad, 2014). In the process of engaging in research through diffractive analysis, I have needed to struggle with blurred and often unclear delineations, sometimes contradictory and inconsistent meetings of phenomena and the multiplicities and pluralities that characterise an assemblage that is enactive and dynamic, rather than static and passive. Lenz Taguchi and Palmer (2013) describe diffractive analysis as

> an enactment of flows of differences, where differences get made in the process of reading data into each other and identifying what diffractive patterns emerge in these readings.
>
> (676)

Davies (2021) reminds us of the unpredictable nature of diffractive research processes that can be both confronting and unsettling but that are, at the same time, exciting and effective in stimulating new ways of thinking. As I have explained in a previous publication (Frizell, 2023), it took me time to grasp the idea of working with diffractive meeting places of differences, rather than the differences themselves. I spent time on a beach, standing in a blustery wind, watching waves bending and spreading as they encountered obstructions in meeting places that always created something new.

Research, within this ethico-onto-epistemological paradigm, never stands still; it is always in praxis and, as such, lends itself well to research that is practice-led, or practice-as-research (PaR) that brings an immersion within the practice, rather than engaging in a process of stepping outside the subject matter to observe, analyse and measure. This certainly sounds like a cue for improvisational dance as research.

Research through dance improvisation

Improvisational dance practice as research involves a dialogic process between the first-hand immersion in the practice itself and the critical discourses that help the research to challenge and question the practice. This critical eye is essential in

> the creation of new concepts, or navigational tools to help us through the complexities of the *present*, with special focus on the project of *actualizing* the virtual.
>
> (Braidotti, 2019a: 37)

This focus on the relationship between the present and the actualisation of the virtual is a diffractive meeting of past, present and future, as existing knowledge is confronted by knowledge that awaits discovery. This dialogue feeds back into practice. The process has no end point; however, researchers are required to produce outputs (for example, a journal publication, a film, a presentation and a performance) and a punctuation point (deadline) of some kind needs to be agreed. This punctuation point calls for a tangible output that represents the stories-so-far of the inquiry. Outputs are vital as part of a wider dialogic research process in the professional field and, as such, will contribute to ongoing professional discourses. Conclusions, however, are rarely finite.

PaR through improvisational dancing bodies provides a frame for the immersion of the researcher in the creativity and contingent nature of movement through play and exploration. For example,

> *Finding myself standing in a movement space, I twist my spine, allowing my arms to follow the flow of the twist, without a preconceived idea of where this movement will lead. I trust that as my head gently pulls me out of the twist and my arm punctuates the movement by lifting in front of my chest, I am treading new ground that weaves poetically into unknown territory.*

On another occasion, whilst engaged in non-stylised, environmental movement on the wilds of Dartmoor in South West UK, I recall how

> I closed my eyes and rested my head on a ledge, wrapping my arms around the rock. I became acutely conscious of how I was placing my body in the space, against the solid surface.
>
> (Frizell, 2020: 218)

These encounters with the world become the affective flows of material bodies as my experience of improvisational dance folds into the material world. In *Interruption 5: Coming down to earth* (Pages 97–99) that precedes this chapter,

I describe an experience of this folding into the material world. In these moments, I am engaging in a process of worlding (Manning, 2012). These worlding relations are key to improvisational dance as a way of thinking into and through the world with the moving body. As I do so, I defamiliarise myself with the anthropocentrism of my experience; that is, I cut across the exceptionalism that separates human from other-than-human. My movement becomes part of an embodied, embedded material-affective flow.

Working with improvised movement through, for example, live or filmed performance, either indoors or outdoors in the landscape, engages 'materially creative thinking within and through the practices of dance making' (Midgelow, 2021: 112). Improvisational dance as research provides an opportunity to turn towards the dynamic, contingent nature of moving bodies, which are always in the process of becoming within the affective economy of rhizomatic assemblages. Bacon (2010, 2020) emphasises the processual nature of PaR and dance improvisation as a modality to generate knowledge is well documented, for example, Ashley (2016, 2019), Bacon (2010, 2017, 2020), Barbour (2018), Blockmans et al. (2020), Chodorow (1999), Fraleigh (2019), Frizell (2012, 2014, 2017, 2020, 2023), Hayes (2013), Kramer (2012, 2015), LaMothe (2015, 2018, 2020), Manning (2012), Markula (2006), McDowall (2019), Midgelow (2021), Phelan (1993), Rova (2017, 2023), Sheets-Johnstone (2011), Stromsted (2015) and Trimingham (2002). Hayes (2013) considers that the kinaesthetic empathy of practice is itself an emergent research method, enabling the researcher to connect relationally to the intra-subjective space of existence. This makes visible multiply entangled encounters that are experienced through movement in any one moment, calling upon 'spontaneity, resilience, presence, adaption, readiness, responsiveness, risk, and willingness' (Fraleigh, 2019: 67).

Researching beyond conclusions

It is important that, as practitioners, we sustain our own curiosity through research inquiry and, similarly as researchers, that we ground our inquiry in practice. My own journey in terms of what research does and how it can be done has shifted over the years though qualitative methodologies, including case-study, auto-ethnography, interpretive phenomenological analysis (IPA) (Smith et al., 2012) and PaR (Midgelow, 2021), for postqualitative inquiry (Murris, 2021, Lather & St Pierre, 2013, St Pierre, 2014). In my experience, research has been a potent process of renewing my thoughts about ways of being in the world, ways of thinking about what constitutes knowledge and ways of developing my practice as a therapist, supervisor, artist and educator. Research has also enabled me to add to the diverse knowledge base of professional fields that include the arts therapies, ecologically informed psychotherapeutic practices and critical disability studies. Throughout that research, I have been loyal to the primacy of relational, creative moving bodies of all kin(ds) whilst also remaining committed to critical discourses that support a reframing and reconceptualising of the ways in which we think about that experience.

The entangled tensions of material-discursive research practices bring a richness to postqualitative research, staying with ethico-onto-epistemological contradictions and dynamics, rather than finding methodological frameworks within which research needs to fit. That is not to say that methodological frameworks are not useful containers that can help us shape research; however, the method itself needs to be held lightly and responsively. Postqualitative research has the potential to challenge cultural norms and decentre humans as exclusive makers of meaning, supporting researchers to question the attachments that 'keep us from thinking and living differently' (Lather & St. Pierre, 2013: 631).

Arguably, I might consider that practitioners are all researchers who seek to create new knowledge and insights about their practice. The question of how practice becomes research and research becomes practice opens debates about intention, consent and ethical parameters. My practice as a therapist is itself an inquiry into a transformative relational process and, as such, I am constantly inquiring into optimising my understanding, skills and ethics of the professional services that I deliver. Researching, in this sense, is (arguably) always happening. Or perhaps what I am describing might just be considered good practice, rather than research. I wonder what you, the reader, think about this.

As I began this chapter, a colleague sent me a despondent email saying that they were feeling *horribly hopeless about research*. I received this sentiment as a provocation to think about what research means, what research does and the nature of generating innovative ways of knowing and becoming with the world. I also resonate with that horrible hopelessness in relation to research, particularly at times when I cannot seem to access my capacity to bring to life anything new, anything meaningful and anything worthwhile into the world of knowledge creation. Within a university context, a competitive research ranking might favour positivist research that generates data that can be counted and measured. At the same time, academics' workloads have intensified to such an extent that it is hard to find critical thinking spaces for material-discursive processes that are less easy to count. Universities are competitively ranked, and in the process of gathering a body of research to submit, the research that counts will often be the research outcomes that can *be* counted and that are seen to have an immediate impact in their application and influence in policy and practice. As universities are competitively and publicly ranked, so too are the academics producing the research, each being given points corresponding to the value of their respective outputs in relation to wider institutional requirements. These points are then linked to promotion opportunities, creating an atmosphere in which it is hard for young academics who need a secure career to support them in their working lives, to deviate from the wave of positivist principles.

The email from my colleague reminds me that in those moments of feeling horribly hopeless, it can be helpful to reach out and share that vulnerability with other trusted researchers (most of whom will also know that place), finding a place of solidarity. There is also a *horrible hopelessness* in the world as the climate emergency quickens and as social, economic, political and environmental inequalities become acutely apparent. As researchers, we have an opportunity to generate inquiry that develops and fosters empathic, creative ways of moving through this world that are ethically, ontologically and epistemologically anti-oppressive. Postqualitative research, which includes ecofeminist, posthuman and new materialist ideas, challenges the ways particular kinds of knowledge become privileged, decolonising processes that have entrapped other-than-verbal investigations in the margins, banished the otherwise enabled to a place of subordination and subjected the material world to a place of objectification. The challenge is to practise research that seeks 'to re-orient thought to experiment and create new forms of thought and life' (St Pierre, 2021: 163).

I hope that this chapter will offer you provocations to think about your own unique contribution to the different ways that knowledge can emerge.

Provocation

I invite you to bring your focus to your own relationship with research inquiry. What does it mean to you?

Using a creative art form (for example, dance, music, art, poetry, story, photography and role play), spend some time free associating with the question through the art form. Just let it take you wherever it needs to go.

Taking what you have created as a starting point, spend some time alone or with a peer/colleague, reflecting on how your creative response is suggestive of what research inquiry means to you.

Notes

1 Barad's neologism ethico-onto-epistemology (Barad, 2007) (i.e., the way justice is thought about and applied, the nature of existing in the world and the parameters within which knowledge emerges) brings a new materialist lens of multiplicity and diversity to postqualitative inquiry.
2 For Mental Capacity Act 2005, see: www.legislation.gov.uk/ukpga/2005/9/section/33
3 For further information on David Woodger, see: www.gold.ac.uk/stacs/staff/woodger-david/
4 See '(t)hing power' (Bennett, 2010: 20) explained in Chapter 1.
5 Thank you Helen Poynor for this play on words in conversation.
6 Deleuze and Guattari (1987) suggest that: 'The BwO is what remains when you take everything away. What you take away is precisely the phantasy, and significances and subjectifications as a whole' (151).

References

Ashley, T. (2016). Embodiment and digital interactivity: Towards posthuman somatic practices. *Journal of Dance and Somatic Practices*, Vol. 8, No. 1, pp. 3–9.

Ashley, T. (2019). Improvisation and the earth: Dancing in the moment as ecological practice. In L. Midgelow (ed.), *The Oxford Handbook of Improvisation in Dance*, pp. 595–610. New York: Oxford University Press.

Bacon, J. (2010). The voice of her body: Somatic practices as a basis for creative research methodology. *Journal of Dance and Somatic Practices*. Vol. 2, No. 1, pp. 63–74.

Bacon, J. (2017). Authentic movement as a practice for wellbeing. In V. Karkou, S. Oliver and S. Lycouris (eds.), *The Oxford Handbook of Dance and Wellbeing*, pp. 149–164. Oxford: Oxford University Press.

Bacon, J. (2020). Informed by the goddess: Explicating a processual methodology. In A. Williamson and B. Sellers-Young (eds.), *Spiritual Herstories: Call of the Soul in Dance Research*, pp. 69–87. Bristol: Intellect.

Barad, K. (2007). *Meeting the Universe Halfway: Quantum Physics and the Entanglement of Matter and Meaning*. London: Duke University Press.

Barad, K. (2012). On touching – the inhuman that therefore I am. *Differences*, Vol. 23, No. 3, pp. 206–223.

Barad, K. (2014). Diffracting diffraction: Cutting together-apart. *Parallax*, Vol. 20, No. 3, pp. 168–187.

Barbour, K. (2018). Dancing epistemology. Situating feminist analysis. In S. Fraleigh (ed.), *Back to the Dance Itself: Phenomenologies of the Body in Performance*, pp. 233–246. California, CA: Illinois.

Bennett, J. (2010). *Vibrant Matter: A Political Ecology of Things*. Durham: Duke University Press.

Blockmans, I., De Schauwer, E., Van Hove, G. and Enzlin, P. (2020). Retouching and revisiting the strangers within: An exploration journey on the waves of meaning and matter in dance. *Qualitative Inquiry*, Vol. 26, No. 7, pp. 733–742.

Braidotti, R. (2019a). A theoretical framework for the critical posthumanities. *Theory, Culture and Society*. Vol. 36, No. 6, pp. 31–61.

Chodorow, J. (1999). Dance therapy and the transcendent function. In P. Pallaro (ed.), *Authentic Movement: Essays by Mary Starks Whitehouse, Janet Adler and Joan Chodorow*, pp. 236–252. London: Jessica Kingsley.

Davies, B. (2014). Reading anger in early childhood intra-actions: A diffractive analysis. *Qualitative Inquiry*, Vol. 20, No. 6, pp. 734–741.

Davies, B. (2021). *Entanglement in the World's Becoming and the Doing of New Materialist Inquiry*. New York: Routledge.

Deleuze, G. and Guattari, F. (1987). *A Thousand Plateaus: Capitalism and Schizophrenia*. London: Continuum.

Fox, N. and Alldred, P. (2015). New materialist social inquiry: Designs, methods and the research-assemblage. *International Journal of Social Research Methodology*, Vol. 18, No. 4, pp. 399–414.

Fraleigh, S. (2019). A philosophy of the improvisational body. In L. Midgelow (ed.), *The Oxford Handbook of Improvisation in Dance*, pp. 65–88. New York: Oxford University Press.

Frizell, C. (2012). Embodiment and the supervisory task. *Body, Movement and Dance in Psychotherapy: An International Journal for Theory, Research and Practice*, Vol. 7, No. 4, pp. 293–304.

Frizell, C. (2014). Discovering the language of the ecological body. *Self and Society: An International Journal for Humanistic Psychology*, Vol. 41, No. 4, pp. 15–21.

Frizell, C. (2017). Entering the world: Dance movement psychotherapy and the complexity of beginnings with learning disabled clients. In G. Unkovich, C. Buttee and J. Butler (eds.), *Dance Movement Psychotherapy with People with Learning Disabilities: Out of the Shadows, into the Light*, pp. 9–21. Abingdon: Routledge.

Frizell, C. (2020). Reclaiming our innate vitality: Bringing embodied narratives to life through dance movement psychotherapy. In A. Williamson and B. Sellers-Young (eds.), *Spiritual Herstories: Call of the Soul in Dance Research*, pp. 207–220. Bristol: Intellect.

Frizell, C. (2023). The cat, the foal and other meetings that make a difference: Posthuman research that reanimates our responsiveness to knowing and becoming. In C. Frizell and M. Rova (eds.), *Creative Bodies in Therapy, Performance and Community Research and Practice that Brings Us Home*, pp. 50–61. London: Routledge.

Frizell, C. and Woodger, D. (2019). Removing the threat of exclusion in schools: Creating inclusive educational environments. *Youth and Policy*, pp. 1–8 (ISNN 0262–9798).

Goldsmith, L. and Skirton, H. (2015). Research involving people with a learning disability – methodological challenges and ethical considerations. *Journal of Research in Nursing*, Vol. 20, No. 6, pp. 435–446.

Hayes, J. (2013). *Soul and Spirit in Dance Movement Psychotherapy: A Transpersonal Approach*. London: Jessica Kingsley.

Kramer, P. (2012). Bodies, Rivers, Rocks and Trees: Meeting agentic materiality in contemporary outdoor dance practices. *Performance Research*, Vol. 17, No. 4, pp. 83–91.

Kramer, P. (2015). *Dancing Materiality: A Study of Agency and Confederations in Contemporary Outdoor Dance Practices*. Unpublished PhD thesis. Coventry: Coventry University.

LaMothe, K. (2015). *Why We Dance: A Philosophy of Bodily Becoming*. New York: Columbia University Press.

LaMothe, K. (2018). As the earth dances: A philosophy of bodily becoming. In S. Fraleigh (ed.), *Back to the Dance Itself: Phenomenologies of the Body in Performance*. Chicago: University of Illinois Press.

LaMothe, K. (2020). Writing why we dance: The predicament, pitfalls, potential and promise of writing about dance and spirituality. In A. Williamson and B. Sellers-Young (eds.), *Spiritual Herstories: Call of the Soul in Dance Research*, pp. 393–413. Bristol: Intellect.

Lather, P. (2013). Methodology-21: What do we do in the afterward? *International Journal of Qualitative Studies in Education*, Vol. 26, No. 6, pp. 634–645.

Lather, P. and St. Pierre, E. (2013). Post-qualitative research. *International Journal of Qualitative Studies in Education*, Vol. 26, No. 6, pp. 629–633.

Lenz Taguchi, H. and Palmer, A. (2013). A more 'liveable' school? A diffractive analysis of the performative enactments of girls' ill-/well-being with(in) school environments. *Gender and Education*, Vol. 25, No. 6, pp. 671–687.

Linnell, S. (2006). *Towards Ethical " Arts of Existence": Through Art Therapy and Narrative Therapy*. Unpublished thesis. Western Sydney: University of Western Sydney College of Arts.

MacDonald, S. and Wiens, B. (2019). Mobilizing the "multimangle": Why new materialist research methods in public participatory art matter. *Leisure Sciences*, Vol. 41, No. 5, pp. 366–384.

MacLure, M. (2010). The offence of theory. *Journal of Education Policy*, Vol. 25, No. 2, pp. 277–286.

Manning, E. (2012). *Always More Than One: Individuation's Dance*. Durham: Duke University Press.

Markula, P. (2006). The dancing body without organs: deleuze, femininity, and performing research. *Qualitative Inquiry*, Vol. 12, No. 1, pp. 3–27.

McDowall, L. (2019). Exploring uncertainties of language in dance Improvisation. In L. Midgelow (ed.), *The Oxford Handbook of Improvisation in Dance*. New York: Oxford University Press.

McLeod, J. (2001). *Qualitative Research in Counselling and Psychotherapy*. London: Sage.

Midgelow, V. (2021). Practice-as-research. In S. Dodds (ed.), *The Bloomsbury Companion to Dance Studies*, pp. 111–144. London: Bloomsbury.

Murris, K. (ed.). (2021). Making kin: Postqualitative, new materialist and posthumanist research. In Murris, K. (ed.), *Navigating the Postqualitative, New Materialist and Critical Posthumanist Terrain across Disciplines: An Introductory Guide*, pp. 1–21. Oxon: Routledge.

Nkanga, O. (2019). Imagining the scars of a Landscape. *Tate. YouTube*: https://youtu.be/qZZruEToDCI

Phelan, P. (1993). *Unmarked*. London: Routledge.

Reason, M. (2012). Photography and the representation of kinesthetic empathy. In D. Reynolds and M. Reason (eds.), *Kinesthetic Empathy in Creative and Cultural Practices*, pp. 237–258. Bristol: Intellect.

Rova, M. (2017). Embodying kinaesthetic empathy through interdisciplinary practice-based research. *The Arts in Psychotherapy*, Vol. 55, pp. 164–173.

Rova, M. (2023). Kinaesthetic entanglements and creative immersion in embodied performance. In C. Frizell and M. Rova (eds.), *Creative Bodies in Therapy, Performance and Community Research and Practice that Brings Us Home*, pp. 36–49. Oxon: Routledge.

Sheets-Johnstone, M. (2011). *The Primacy of Movement*. Philadelphia: John Benjamins Pub. Co.

Skaife, S., Morris, L., Tipple, R. and Velada, D. (2020). The story of the camera, a case study of an art therapy large group. *Group Analysis*, Vol. 53, No. 1, pp. 37–59.

Smith, J., Flowers, P. and Larkin, M. (2012). *Interpretative Phenomenological Analysis*. London: Sage Publications Ltd.

Stewart, K. (2007). *Ordinary Affects*. Durham: Duke University Press Books.

St Pierre, E. (2014). A brief and personal history of postqualitative research toward "Post Inquiry". *Journal of Curriculum Theorizing*, Vol. 30, No. 2, pp. 2–19.

St Pierre, E. (2021). Why postqualitative inquiry? *Qualitative Inquiry*, Vol. 27, No. 2, pp. 163–166.

Stromsted, T. (2015). Authentic movement and the evolution of soul's body® work. *Journal of Dance and Somatic Practices*, Vol. 7, No. 2, pp. 339–357.

Trimingham, M. (2002). A methodology for practice as research. *Studies in Theatre and Performance*, Vol. 22, No. 1, pp. 54–60.

Unkovich, U., Butté, C. and Butler, J. (eds.). (2017). *Dance Movement Psychotherapy with People with Learning Disabilities: Out of the Shadows, into the Light*. Abingdon: Routledge.

Williamson, A. and Sellers-Young, B. (eds.). (2020). *Spiritual Herstories: Call of the Soul in Dance Research*. Bristol: Intellect.

Interruption 6

In the face of the storm

It is 1985. I stand on a Tahitian beach – a 27-year-old hopeful Westerner, surfing the waves of Thatcher's economic revolution. I have flown to New Zealand to teach, taking the opportunity to stop off along the way. As someone who gave up flying at the millennium due to the environmental crisis, with hindsight I wonder why I did not question a long-haul flight to engage in a task that could very easily have been accomplished by someone local.

I look down at my toes in the sand and breathe in the vivid blue of the Pacific Ocean. A wave of discomfort surges in me as I remember that this paradise lies within the Polynesian nuclear test site, an environmental violation lurking invisibly in the materiality of this place. Waves ripple over the fine particles of golden sand glistening on my ankles.

I slip my sandals back on and leave the beach to jump on a bus heading out of town to Gauguin's house. Polynesian music blasts from a speaker. I hold the handrail as the bus rattles unevenly from side to side. A middle-aged Tahitian man clothed in a brightly coloured shirt and well-worn, open-toed sandals offers a welcoming smile, revealing two dazzling gold teeth. I avert my eyes involuntarily from this male gaze. He shrugs and strikes up a conversation with another passenger. On adjacent seats, a group of women each clutch a suckling baby to their breast and engage in animated chatter.

I feel out of place as a white-skinned Western woman with cropped hair and a blue cotton dress, clinging to the handrail of the bus and peering wide-eyed out of the window at the road lined with wild orchids, behind which a flush of emerald green sweeps upwards to the plantations on the mountainside. Dark clouds hover at the mountain peaks.

I alight at Gauguin's house and inside, find myself immersed in the vibrancy of the paintings. Leaving the house, I walk back to the road. In an instant, clouds sweep overhead, and a torrent of rain soaks me to the skin, flattening my blue cotton dress to my body. Flashes of lightning light the silver-black sky. Thunder roars and giant balls of rain ricochet off the steaming ground in a cacophony of sound. I open my arms, feeling alive in the face of this tropical storm.

More than a decade later, I sit opposite my new therapist in her consulting room. Next to the glowing wood burner is a box of matches and on the front

DOI: 10.4324/9781003322658-13

of the box is a small print of one of Gauguin's paintings that I have seen hanging in his Tahitian house. The picture takes me back to my experience of that moment. I remember feeling so out of place. I remember the contradictions of a paradise that had been polluted by invisible radiation. I remember my sense of powerlessness and aliveness in the face of the storm.

7 Practising as a craft

Maeve knocks on the door and walks quickly across the floor to join me. She is wearing a light blue headscarf and as she sits down, she brushes it back with her right hand to reveal her bald head. I am taken aback at this sudden and unexpected hair loss.

'I shaved my head in solidarity with a friend who has cancer,' She says quickly.

I put my right hand on my chest.

'Gosh,' I say, my face crumpling involuntarily.
   'I wanted her to know I was by her side . . . if you know what I mean,' She says.

Maeve pulls the scarf back over her head and throws the corner across her right shoulder to drape down her back. She averts her eyes. I look down, noticing her odd socks, one purple with yellow stripes running across the instep and the other dark blue with black dots. There's a tenderness in my stomach as I lower my hand to place it gently on top of my left hand resting on my lap.

'I feel like I need to be close to the ground,' Maeve points across the room.
   'Shall we sit on those cushions?' she suggests.
   'OK,' I nod.

As we shift position, heavy rain drums on the roof. I sit on a cushion and Maeve remains standing. The rain stops as suddenly as it began. Clasping my arms around my knees, I look up at Maeve. Our gaze locks in the silence. I feel small and vulnerable, as if cowering at the feet of a

DOI: 10.4324/9781003322658-14

giant. We continue to return each other's gaze and I try to formulate something to say. Nothing comes.

Maeve takes a breath,

'Actually, I hope you don't mind, but I'm going to lie on the floor.'

Maeve lies on her back and her headscarf falls to the floor. I wait, intrigued by what is unfolding, aware that she is now at *my* feet. A lighter shower of rain patters on the roof. I notice a thin layer of dust on the gato drum at the other side of the studio. Maeve lifts the palms of her hands to cover her head and, facing away from me, slowly contracts her body into a foetal position. She remains there and I notice the curve of her back, the soles of her brightly patterned socks tucked up beneath her body and her fingertips clasped around the smooth bare skin of her skull. The rain continues. I feel a well of grief rising through my stomach, into the back of my throat and up through my jaw. The light in the studio dims and out of the window, the sky has turned petrol blue. There is a distant rumble of thunder. My hands are clutched tightly around my knees, and in my mind's eye, I scoop Maeve up into my arms and cradle her as I might a baby. I loosen my grip around my knees and feel my shoulders drop.

Maeve slowly unfurls onto her back, stretching her arms out along the floor to make a long line between her fingertips and toes. I release my arms and rest my hands on either side of my torso on the rough woven surface of the Moroccan cushion cover. Maeve begins to roll slowly away from me, tipping onto her right side to face the floor and then returning to lie on her back, opening out her right arm on a diagonal trajectory. Leaving her scarf where it falls, she continues this sequential rolling, as if in slow motion, over and over until she reaches the other end of the studio. Lying face down, Maeve presses the palms of her hands into the floor and pushes herself up to kneel, silhouetted at the other end of the room. The rain stops, and the sun throws a shaft of light across the blue scarf that lies abandoned between us. Maeve turns her face towards the illuminated scarf and then looks at me, bringing her body round to sit cross-legged, hands cupped around her knees.

I slide off my cushion to feel the cool wooden floor beneath me to mirror her position on the other side of the room. Maeve's scarf remains discarded on the floor between us. The shaft of light disappears behind the clouds.

Looking directly at each other, we smile.

Maeve looks down.

Practising in rhizomatic assemblages

Maeve and I had arrived in this place of diffractive potential, facing each other, cross-legged on the floor, both immersed in this unique unfolding of relational experience. I wonder how you, the reader, might have responded. Might you have waited for Maeve's next move? Made a punctuating statement of observation? Invited verbal reflection on this arrival? Every intervention is situated within a complex, rhizomatic, material-discursive convergence of the present moment, and there is no formula for how any one of us might respond. Practitioner Poynor (2023) reminds us that

> (b)ecause we are working in the present, in the presence of living beings, moving bodies and feelings, in a live creative process, our response, however considered and theoretically informed, needs to incorporate our own aliveness and a degree of spontaneity if we are to genuinely connect with the experience of the person or group before us.
>
> (101)

As I responded to Maeve, I straddled the emergent diffractive meeting places of theoretically informed positioning and my own spontaneous, relational aliveness. In all professional practising, I am continuously arriving and departing, responding to the unique constellation of any given moment. I do this through material-discursive relationships; through embodied, embedded theoretical perspectives; through emotional, intuitive and sensory flows of the experience; through the phase of the therapy; through emergent narratives and through wider socio-political landscapes. In this vignette, I used few words as we navigated the terrains of a landscape that was created from living, breathing, moving bodies amongst the materiality of matter in time and space, as well as from the explicit narratives that Maeve was bringing, such as gender, illness, compassion and solidarity. At the point at which this vignette is paused, we were sitting facing each other – woman to woman, therapist to client – bodies amongst material bodies, situated spatially, temporally and discursively.

Practising through spacetimematter

As Maeve entered this session, I had initially felt a surge of warmth, and on reflection, I realised how her arrivals had changed over time. When Maeve had begun attending therapy, her entrance had been tentative and apologetic. The session presented here was at least three quarters of the way through our agreed process together, and Maeve seemed to have begun to trust her own significance within an assemblage of *spacetimemattering* situated in unfolding dynamic, relational processes.

Maeve was shifting in her relationship with me as well as with the wider world. Together, we were creating a particular culture, and I had needed to allow Maeve to discover and unpack a painful sense of her own insignificance, rather than being too quick to respond to my impulse to reassure, which can be a counter-transferential avoidance of the client's unbearable anxiety (Casement, 1985). At times, this had been an uncomfortable projection for me to hold, and some weeks prior to the vignette described above, Maeve had brought a dream, which emerged as a transformational gift with regard to exploring the less conscious relational power dynamics. Maeve placed a notebook on her lap, and, opening it, she read out loud:

> *I am in a workshop run by a woman in her 50s or 60s who clearly knows what she's doing. In the background is a man, and every now and again he places his face near me, and I feel scared. I'm excited about attending the workshop, but when I arrive, they ask me to look after the children in a plastic area, away from the adults. I don't want to, but I comply. The plastic construction falls in on the babies, who become puppies, eating plastic bits from a bowl. I want to be with the adults, but I stay where I am, because that's where the woman has put me.*

Practising (as) resistance

When we explored this dream, we found many layers, including a powerful transference at play between us in Maeve's feelings of infantilisation and disempowerment. We explored the man in the background on many levels, including the power dynamics that emerged in the transference and as a patriarchal representation in relation to Maeve's sense of her own worth and entitlement to belong. She linked the image of the plastic-eating puppies in the collapsing enclosure to times in her life when she has experienced her own emotional collapse, as well as linking it to the terror of environmental breakdown. This was a rich dream that helped Maeve link her own personal narratives and her sense of her own agency to our immediate relationship in the room and to the wider narratives of our time in the face of ecological disaster.

We were engaged in a kind of activism through practice (I wondered about calling this practivism) in generating and practising a refusal of patriarchal values in which Maeve had experienced oppression and subordination, through gender, class and her status as a migrant, that were entangled with her unique historical experience of significant relationships. The private and the political are always entangled within the corporeality of the therapeutic assemblages, and therapy can foster a healthy resistance that pushes back at inequalities embedded in the body politic. The term *resistance* in therapy might be used to describe a client who does not respond as we (the professional) might expect or would like. However, I am using the term resistance here as a form of waking up to the ways in which therapy itself can become an act of resistance that enables clients (and therapists) to identify social, political and institutional oppressions that help them think about difficult experiences as, on the one hand, uniquely personal and, on the other hand, symptomatic of wider ideological and institutional malaises.

I found myself profoundly struck by Maeve's act of shaving her head in solidarity with a woman friend who had cancer. The loss of hair, for whatever reason, is significant in any woman's life and I was touched by this radical enactment. Later in the session, Maeve declared that shaving her head felt like an act of defiance. I began wondering to myself about the mythical and symbolic significance of a woman shaving or cutting off the hair on her head as an act of resistance in the face of the oppressions of identity politics, perhaps also linking this enactment to a symbolic expression of our forthcoming separation. The hair on a woman's body holds a complex significance in terms of gender performativity. At around this time, the #MeToo movement was re-surfacing in the media, in response to horrendous acts of misogyny and abuse, and I found myself harbouring powerful associations in relation to gender oppressions that Maeve had disclosed in previous sessions.

Maeve also spoke of the existential anxieties that were provoked by her friend's diagnosis of cancer and spoke of her disturbance at the socio-cultural wall of positivity that served as a defence against thinking about illness and death. Maeve followed the initial unveiling of her shaved head with a rushed explanation to me. I wondered if she was protecting me from the shock and discomfort that she might have anticipated in my response. The scarf seemed to be protecting the world (me) from the shock of her hair loss, from the conversation about cancer, from a symbolic vulnerability and from the existential anxieties that might be provoked. Maeve was stepping into resistance and refusal within the body politic in breaking the spells of gender performativity. I was also struck by my own associations of women wearing headscarves for religious or ideological reasons and as I write this, the wearing and removal of headscarves by women has become increasingly visible as a powerful political statement.

These were all my wonderings that helped me listen to Maeve from the many layers of her direct individual life experience, as well as from the wider discourses around those experiences. In that moment of facing each other cross-legged on the floor at the end of the vignette above, my wonderings and hers constellated and later in the session, we spent time reflecting on the significance of Maeve's enactment in relation to personal and political power.

Practising through less conscious transferential realms

Maeve quickly pulled the scarf back up over her head, and, at her suggestion, we shifted away from the chairs, moving towards the cushions, getting closer to the ground. I then found myself sitting at Maeve's feet and this spatial proximity was a potent statement as I looked up at the woman in the scarf towering above me. Less consciously, perhaps Maeve was playing with power differentials that we had explored through her dream and she quickly changed the spatial relationship from towering over me to lying on the floor at *my* feet. Momentarily, as Maeve towered over me, my thinking seemed to shut down and I have learnt not to defend against these uncomfortable moments when

I am picking up something in the field, something that might be called the countertransference, in which my strong emotional response becomes a vital communication of what is constellating between us. I wondered about my own resonance with *cowering at the feet of giants* as I was drawn into this enactment. Arriving into this particular kind of spatial relationship might not be appropriate with every client, as all therapy is situated and every unfolding response requires a sensitivity to the particular assemblage that is arising. For example, in my work in pupil referral units (PRUs), I was differently cautious of such physical and spatial proximities and would have been careful not to place myself in this vulnerable position. The volatility of some clients, as part of the situated assemblage, necessitated specific and ongoing moment-to-moment risk assessment in order to create the necessary physical and emotional safety.

Maeve then changed the spatial relationship between us by dropping to the floor, and some moments later, Maeve curled into a foetal position at *my* feet. At this point, I noticed the urge to cradle her and I experienced a wave of grief. It was as if there was a collision of, firstly, the sadness and grief of Maeve's stories of attachment; secondly, a kinship with wider socio-political and cultural stories of subordinated others who cower in the face of advanced capitalist, patriarchal giants; and, thirdly, the complexity of my own personal stories of attachment that hovered silently in the field. Rather than trying to disentangle myself from that complicated web, I allowed myself an internal space for my own story, whilst remaining alert to what was being created through Maeve's communication in the moment. Perhaps less consciously, she was questioning the level of my commitment to being by her side, as a therapist and as a woman, particularly as we moved towards an ending and this led to an exploration of how Maeve often experienced the process of therapy as painfully exposing.

As time went on, I had found myself deeply touched by our relationship and Maeve seemed increasingly confident that she mattered, here in this space, in my eyes and in the eyes of the world. This confidence had developed slowly and her dream brought to the surface some useful insights in this therapeutic assemblage.

Practising neutrality as a posthuman entanglement

It is rarely useful and possibly detrimental to share explicitly elements of my own story with a client as this potentially adds an unnecessary distraction, collapses the power of the transferential content and dilutes the intensity of what clients are exploring and what is being enacted. However, I do not consider it useful to subscribe to a fixed rule about neutrality but rather respect neutrality as a guiding principle, within the specificity of any given therapeutic assemblage. Simply being present is itself a disclosure, for example, the clothes I wear, the way I speak, my spontaneous responses, my mannerisms and gestures, the studio in which I work and the less conscious enactments into which I get drawn. If, within new materialist and posthuman ethico-onto-epistemologies,

I consider that I am continuously (re)created through my intra-active participation in the world, then any sense of static neutrality is surely an illusion. A posthuman neutrality (perhaps itself a contradiction) holds a space for me to be simultaneously and spontaneously entangled, while also maintaining an ethical and thoughtful clarity about my role in relation to my own process as I monitor what and how I actively bring to the relationship. Within an intra-active ecology in which all phenomena are mutually implicated, continuously affecting and being affected, I recognise that I am fully implicated in this process as I surf the tensions that are created and that unfold in any moment in any session. Maeve's process of becoming as a client and my process of becoming as a therapist constellated in the potential space between us.

In my mind's eye, I played with all kinds of responses and interpretations in relation to being in the room with Maeve, and my wonderings sometimes became useful as subtle prompts (both implicit and explicit) that might create something new between us. For example, when Maeve was exploring her own experience of gender oppression, it was sometimes useful for me to sprinkle in a provocation (lightly) about wider discourses around intersectionality. Sometimes this sprinkling was ignored by Maeve, and at other times, my sprinkling of a thought provided a line of flight that helped Maeve recognise her experience as part of a wider socio-political phenomena, rather than locating the problem in herself as an individual.

Practising (as) crafting

As I recall this session now, I begin to wonder how to explain my practising, which I find more helpful to think about as a verb (to practise: a doing word) rather than a noun (a practice: a thing). As a verb, practising is alive, fluid and dynamic; it moves with, in, out, along and through the intra-active corporeal field, always in a place of becoming and always through the body politic. As a noun, I may be in danger of defining a practice that becomes a pre-existing entity, available to be recreated, leading to formulaic or mechanistic processes.

As practitioners, we learn skillsets and techniques to support our craft. However, the factors crucial to engaging with those skill sets and techniques are the ethics (the application of justice), the ontologies (ideas about *how* we exist in the world) and epistemologies (the nature of knowledge and how it is known), as well as the emotional commitment to and integrity of providing a service that is heartfelt. Our attitudes towards clients shape and are shaped by the kinds of belief systems by which we live, by which we think and by which we perceive the world. In the same way that research methods are only as effective as the kinds of thinking that we use to implement those methods, so practising skills and techniques, in themselves, are of little value without the philosophical, emotional, corporeal, intellectual, playful and psychic integrity of the practitioner.

In that craft of practising, I draw critically on skills underpinned by the theoretical scaffoldings of psychodynamic thinking. For example, it was useful to think about the stories that Maeve brought about past relationships and to consider how these were a symbolic representation of the immediate relationship between her and me in the transference, alerting me to my less conscious countertransference responses. However, I am wary of allowing interpretations to assume the guise of a pre-existing truth. I consider psychodynamic enactments to be part of ever-changing dynamic landscapes, within matrices of multiple material-discursive processes. In this sense, the conceptualisation of internalised objects[1] can be considered manifestations of complex, relational material-discursive processes that locate individuals in an intra-dependent ecology.

Posthuman and new materialist notions of intra-subjectivity move towards rhizomatic assemblages of mutually implicated phenomena that hover on multiple cusps of diffractive possibilities. The vignette at the beginning of this chapter illustrates how, as a therapist, I remain attentive to a rhizomatic assemblage that comprises a range of material-discursive phenomena, all of which have the capacity to affect and be affected. I was keenly attentive to Maeve's process within the materiality of the indoor or outdoor landscape that is part of the experience, for example, the red velvet chairs, the blue scarf, the patterned odd socks, the rain, the thunder, the sunlight, the rough woven surface of the Moroccan cushion cover, the dust on the gato drum and the wooden floor. Rather than filtering out phenomena in the material and environmental contexts, I welcomed them in as part of the affective flow, and sometimes as lines of flight.

In crafting my professional practising, I need to listen carefully to the unique experience particular to the client. For example, I once worked with a young autistic girl who struggled to manage formal, language-based, human-centred environments, such as the classroom, yet she stepped into her own becoming in an outdoor environment. I would find her in the school garden immersed in the soil, fascinated by the roots of trees, exploring their shapes and textures and pathways into the earth (Frizell, 2014). I attempted to make sense of the experience of this client, traversing theoretical notions of subjectivity that helped me facilitate a therapeutic relationship, whilst connecting to the part of her that knew 'instinctively how to speak with the earth' (16). This was a meaningful place of kinship that moved beyond the human realm.

Practising kinship

Kinship is a place of empathic connection with the corporeal, intra-active web of life in which we participate, that is, the 'the florid machinic, organic, and textural entities with which we share the earth and our flesh' (Haraway, 2016: 1). It is a place of potential and a place of solidarity. I can find kinship, for example, when I become aware of the silence through which birds sing and then allow myself to connect with the bird song on a visceral level. I pause in this mo(ve)ment of diffraction, and in this kinetic encounter, creativity has a chance to incubate (Biondo, 2019) and differences have a chance to meet and thread through each other. I wonder which moments of deep connection you can recall that foster those places of kinship.

In my outdoor work with Kim (Frizell, 2014), the work took us into the tensions between a desire to live ethically as a subject *of* the world and a less conscious complicity with the socio-political, cultural inscriptions of human exceptionalism. Kim used improvisational movement to explore kinship in open moorland, finding

> ways to straddle the personal, cultural and ecological contradictions in-herent in her desire to live ethically and peacefully with the earth and her inadvertent complicity in the hubris of the human species.
>
> (15)

Similarly, the case study of Hassan (Frizell, 2020) illustrates how an empathic, intra-connection with the earth can be rekindled within the therapeutic pro-cess, towards both personal and planetary healing. Hassan accessed a deeply intra-subjective, embodied connection with the image of the tree, and through this, he was able to regulate his overactive nervous system.

These examples illustrate how kinship with more-than-human matter(s) can be fostered through practising both indoors and outdoors.

Practising in the margins of belonging

New materialist and posthuman principles align with practising that brings the corporeality of creative, moving bodies to the centre of relational processes. As dynamic organisms, we create and simultaneously become created by complex relational experiences that are infused with powerful socio-political and cul-tural inscriptions. Creative moving bodies are processes through which we can begin to wonder about this world and where we, too, are wondered about *by* the world. We begin to find ways to locate ourselves as participants in the un-folding of that world, navigating ways of belonging, or not, on conscious and less conscious levels. The intersections of our social identities are always playing out in the corporeality of this unfolding. The practice principles underpinned by new materialism and posthumanism challenge the hierarchies of anthro-pocentric hubris and foster manifestations of ecological intra-dependence and kinship.

DMP and ecopsychotherapeutic practitioners have historically struggled with professional identity politics. Both professions challenge the parameters of psychotherapy as an indoor, human-centred talking cure, and both profes-sions arguably have grown from the margins of mainstream paradigms. The emphasis on corporeality and ecological awareness resists anthropocentric and Eurocentric values that privilege individuality and language over collec-tive community and material sensibility. In recent years, both modalities have steadily grown in terms of professional visibility and have become increasingly well-established as independent practising and as part of multidisciplinary

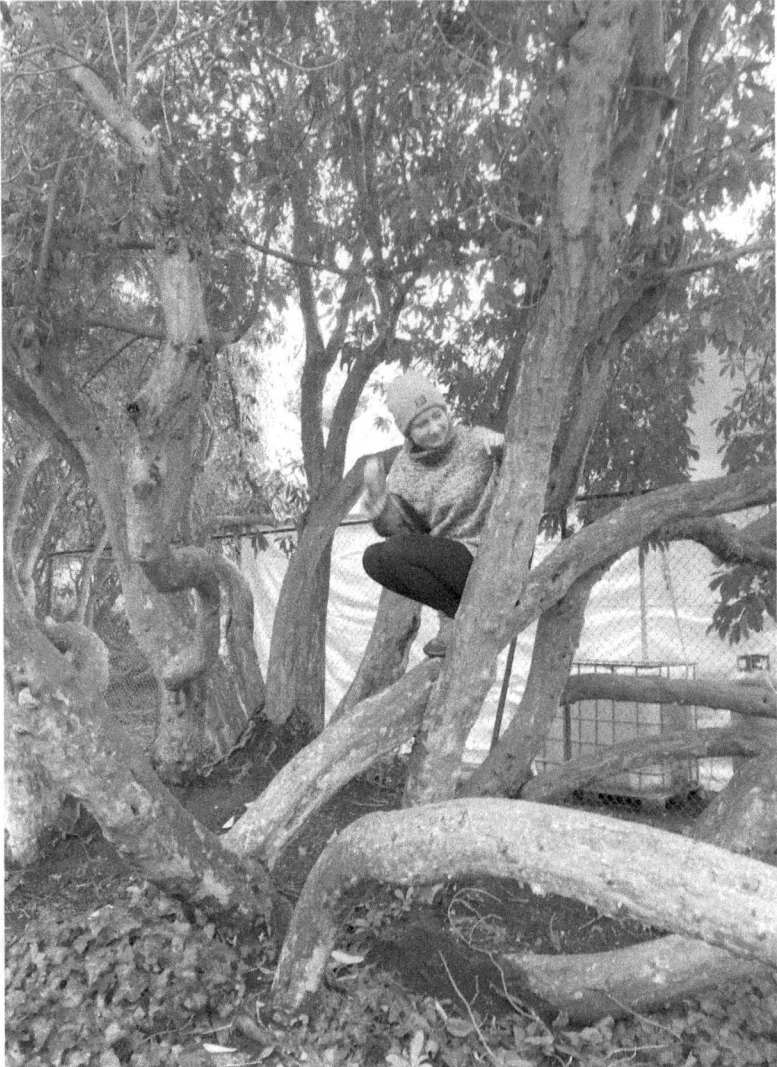

Figure 7.1 Connection.

Source: Photograph by the author.

teams. This evolution has happened despite a political drive for hyper-rational paradigms in psychotherapy that are shaped by a neoliberalist drive to provide quick-fix, solution-focused interventions that measure well-being on scales of one to ten. Neoliberalism, within an advanced capitalist culture, generates systems of (un)care that privilege number-crunching, rational outcome measures over a relational, emotional and soulful delivery of services that find kinship in the craft of practising. Capitalist ideologies are lodged in our care systems, and therapeutic services are often delivered within frameworks of care that demand resource-saving, quick-fix solutions (Brown & Omand, 2022, Dalal, 2018, Skaife & Martyn, 2022).

It is perhaps no coincidence that, as public awareness of the environmental crisis has grown and as inequalities and abuses of power in relation to diverse social identities have become increasingly exposed through the media, it has become clear that we need to find new ways of practising that are relevant to the twenty-first century. Human exceptionalism has given rise to environmental injustices, as well as inequalities that manifest in socio-political, community and institutional systems. Intersectionality, as a practising principle, brings together the identity politics of the material (lived experience) and the discursive (the overlapping discourses implicated in that experience) within rhizomatic assemblages.

Practising (as) inquiry

My own practising as an ecofeminist therapeutic practitioner, educator, facilitator and researcher has evolved through an assemblage of supporting practices that have provided transformative places of inquiry. These include supervision, my own therapy, training courses and continued professional development, peer exchange, reading and study groups, engaging with literature, writing, researching, activism, creative processes indoors and outdoors, as well as just experiencing the world as I meet with the external events of life that provoke entanglements in sometimes unpredictable ways. These are all processes of inquiry that provide opportunities to reconfigure the thoughts that I use to think about the world and the ways in which I engage in professional practising by inviting reflection on *how* I do what I do. These dynamic processes foster my approach as a motivated, enlivened and dynamic practitioner. They help me keep abreast of wider socio-political discourses that shape and are shaped by the situated assemblages in which I work. They guide me into my own affective capacity within material-discursive worlds. They enable me to engage in *worlding*[2] as a practice principle.

Arguably, all practising *is* inquiry, and, in this sense, the boundaries between researching and practising can overlap and become blurred, as inquiry of all kinds fosters new ways of knowledge-ing and experiencing worlds.

Practising (as) listening

The parent of a learning-disabled child once told me how much she valued having someone listen to her child and witness their experience, without trying to improve them or change them in any way. She reminded me of how powerful it can be simply to be witnessed and experienced by another person, without demanding that the individual be anything other than who they are. Bion (2007) called for psychotherapists to suspend memory, desire and understanding in the process of listening, that is, to put aside the preconceptions that we have about clients and to put aside our desire about who or what they should become and, instead, to become fully present to the experiential communication in the moment. It seems to me that Bion was advocating a capacity for a complexly textured kind of listening and thinking that can become obscured by the desire to do, to produce, to find meaning and to be effective.

I remember working with a group of autistic children in a special school who pushed every boundary imaginable and made the adults around them feel out of control and unable to think. I found myself becoming sucked into the chaos and, at the time, was co-working with a newly qualified practitioner who was keen to use all the newly acquired strategies from their specialist autism training. We thought about whether we were not being structured enough or being too structured. We considered to what extent we should tolerate chaos within safe boundaries or perhaps we should bring in a zero-tolerance strategy. We wondered if this was about individual children. Or the staff. Or the school. Or the autism. Or us. Did we need more supervision? I was being sucked into the very chaos that was manifesting in the expression of these children in their acting out, preventing me from listening to, and thinking about the communication.

In the midst of this, I had a dream in which I was sitting on a bench balanced on the edge of a cliff. When I realised the precarity of this position, I began to panic; one false move would mean certain death. I woke with a sense of terror in my fast-beating heart and quickening breath. The brief image in the dream embodied a dilemma, the outcome of which was seemingly out of my control. I reflected on this dream with an intuitive sense of its significance, particularly in relation to my imaginal experience of this tipping point and the palpable terror that I had felt. I thought about how the climate emergency balances on a precarious edge as we try to continue with business as usual.

When I next returned to the school, I shared my dream to my colleague, who had conscientiously been reading up on autism and dissociation, on Melanie Klein's splitting and on chaos theory, whilst also urgently booking extra supervision sessions. Linking our thinking to psychodynamic theories, we also let our reflections sink into the wider implications of a world out of balance. This group of children were enacting an unbearable precarity, and the dream helped me realise how I was so caught up in trying to solve the problem of the chaos (the symptom) that I had lost the capacity to listen to and to think about the underlying less conscious communication of deep distress on local and collective levels. In trying to find a solution, I had been sucked into the chaos. Through the dream, I was more able to realise the emotional resonance of the helplessness and hopelessness being communicated on a worlding, bodied level. I invited my colleague into movement improvisation that enabled us to connect kinaesthetically to a place that was more empathic and open, rather than defensive and closed. We were then more able to hold a balance in our work with the children that comprised clear lines of physical and emotional safety, along with an empathic connection with the distress that was being expressed and a stronger capacity to be with and contain the terror and to give it voice so that it could be thought about. We also worked hard at an organisational level with staff to help them also process the stressful pressures within which they were working. This was a collective task of rebalancing and learning to be with, and creating safety within the contradictions, rather than acting on a specific problem to be solved.

In this listening, we can discover those diffractive meeting places that create new insights.

Practising through diffractions

In practice, diffractive meeting places are moments of potential transformation as illustrated in the following account of my work with Clive, a 10-year-old boy in a PRU. He was rigid in his thinking and easily upset by changes in routine. Clive was highly articulate but prone to lashing out in uncontrollable tantrums when distressed. When he was referred to me, Clive had been at the PRU for over a year after being excluded from school due to disruptive behaviour.

Initially I was struck by Clive's small stature, his alert attention and his adult-like conversation. Clive maintained a clear spatial distance between himself and me and I noticed that I tended to feel empty and stuck in my initial contact with him. In the first session, Clive wandered about the room unable to settle, saying that he felt lost. I thought that I might contain his apparent anxiety with some structure; however, my suggestions were immediately rejected with hyper-rational reasoning about unsuitability. For example, in response to my reflection that it was hard to begin and that he might like to tell me something about himself, he said that he shouldn't need to do that because I should have read his notes and everything that I needed to know would be there. Fair point, I thought to myself, noticing that I felt awkward and slightly hurt. As I reflected on how I might respond, Clive jumped up and initiated a movement pattern. This involved a continuous trotting to a regular rhythm, whilst individual body parts moved in isolation of each other. As he moved, he threw out instructions such as,

'So, you can turn your head and legs in any direction, but you must keep your torso facing the front wall.'

I was intrigued by the juxtapositioning of simultaneously differently moving body parts. The moving body took on a whole new dimension for me, and as I watched, I was reminded of attending a Steve Paxton[3] workshop many years before in which I was challenged to move with relational restrictions on different parts of the body, such as performing a movement score with my leg remaining connected to another dancer. Clive's moving body made me feel uncomfortable and aesthetically inspired at the same time. The discomfort resided in the rigid rules imposed on the moving body, and the aesthetic inspiration arose from witnessing such a different and unique way of moving.

Clive and I were meeting weekly for 45-minute sessions. During the first few weeks, he would engage in similar spontaneous improvisations, creating rules that both restricted and opened up new possibilities. The sequences then began to involve complex plots, which included themes of being pursued, getting stuck and being rescued. On one occasion, he was travelling through an imaginary river, fleeing from the enemy. The water turned to ice, and Clive became stuck. He held a frozen position, lying on his back with his upper back supported by his elbows. He looked tense and distressed. He called me over, telling me to melt the ice around his elbows and feet. I approached him and joined the enactment, holding the palms of my hands towards his elbows, saying,

'Here comes the warmth.'

As I did so, his body became fluid and relaxed, and he crawled towards the place in which I had been sitting. I joined him, noticing that he was more able to tolerate a closer distance between us. Clive was then able to think about the stuck frozen bit inside him. He acknowledged that he often found the world a hostile place.

Towards the end of our work together, Clive initiated an improvisation in which he was in a dark forest. He walked with jerky movements, his body tense and alert. He bumped into a tree and fell, hurt, his body becoming limp and lifeless. He then began to pull himself along, commando crawling through the undergrowth. He found himself in a swamp and asked me to throw him a line to pull him out. I approached the edge of the imaginary swamp and threw him an imaginary rope that he grabbed, and I pulled him to shore. He clambered out of the swamp and lay on his back, staring at the ceiling. He began to talk about how lonely he felt, and how he would like to go back to mainstream school as he craved friendships with children of his own age. These embodied improvisations that had become part of our work together seemed to be enabling Clive to imagine different narratives within permissive, rather than hostile, environments. I was increasingly moved by the ways in which Clive was able to allow improvisational movement and imaginative play to enable narratives to unfold, and he was increasingly able to reflect on these.

Practising (in)conclusions

In this chapter, I have animated some of the ideas about practising in the diffractive meeting places of ecofeminist DMP and ecopsychotherapy, referencing posthumanism, new materialism and the critical discourses of intersectionality. The transdisciplinary nature of these practices provides opportunities to problematise the professions that practitioners are trying to create and, at the same time, by which practitioners are created. The professional *we* is troubled in the quest to find this identity.

I have selected elements of my practising to give you some insight into the ways that I bring together a range of practice principles, within the idea of developing practising as an active, dynamic verb, rather than a noun. The starting point for practising is always being present to my own experience. Through empathic listening, I track my own emotional, conceptual, intuitive, imaginative and bodied mo(ve)ment-to-mo(ve)ment presence in relation to the client(s) as part of the wider assemblage of phenomena.

Practitioners rightly seek to earn a living from their valuable work, and they do so within turbulent and competitive professional waters within a dominant context of hyper-rationality and managerialism (Brown & Omand, 2022, Dalal, 2018, Skaife & Martyn, 2022) as well as within the deregulation of care services (Weintrobe, 2021). The inherent transdisciplinarity of ecofeminist DMP practice and ecopsychotherapy, along with the critical discourses of new materialism, posthumanism and intersectionality, enables practitioners to resist and refuse powerful positivist and dominant discourses and move into alternative ways of being in the world. As practitioners enter the lived experience of practice and research with emotional connectivity, creativity, spontaneity and intuition, the (sometimes) abstract critical discourses are vital in maintaining practice that is critically fluid and accountable.

Provocation

Reflecting on your role as a practitioner, how might you describe your craft and what it is that makes it uniquely yours?

Notes

1 The term *internalised objects* is derived from a psychoanalytic school of thought about object relations, by which representations of significant early attachments inform patterns of relating.
2 *Worlding* is a term coined by Erin Manning (2014) to describe a corporeal, immersive experience in the wonderment of the world.
3 Steve Paxton pioneered innovative dance and choreography by challenging ideas about dance, performance and the ways bodies move.

References

Bion, W. (2007). (Fifth edition. First published 1970) *Attention and Interpretation*. London: Karnac.

Biondo, J. (2019). Stillness in dance/movement therapy: Potentiating creativity on the edge and in the void. *American Journal of Dance Therapy*, Vol. 41, No. 1, pp. 113–121.

Brown, C. and Omand, H. (eds.). (2022). *Contemporary Practice in Studio Art Therapy*. London: Routledge.

Casement, P. (1985). *On Learning from the Patient*. London: Routledge.

Dalal, F. (2018). *The Cognitive Behavioural Tsunami: Managerialism, Politics and the Corruption of Science*. Oxon: Routledge.

Frizell, C. (2014). Discovering the language of the ecological body. *Self and Society: An International Journal for Humanistic Psychology*, Vol. 41, No. 4, pp. 15–21.

Frizell, C. (2020). Reclaiming our innate vitality: Bringing embodied narratives to life through dance movement psychotherapy. In A. Williamson and B. Sellers-Young (eds.), *Spiritual Herstories: Call of the Soul in Dance Research*, pp. 207–220. Bristol: Intellect.

Haraway, D. (2016). *Staying with the Trouble*. London: Duke University Press.

Manning, E. (2014). Wondering the world directly – or, how movement outruns the subject. *Body and Society*, Vol. 20, Nos. 3–4, pp. 162–188.

Poynor, H. (2023). Is that yoga or are you just making it up?. In C. Frizell and M. Rova (eds.), *Creative Bodies in Therapy, Performance and Community Research and Practice that Brings Us Home*, pp. 101–108. London: Routledge.

Skaife, S. and Martyn, J. (2022). *Art Psychotherapy Groups in the Hostile Environment of Neoliberalism*. London: Routledge.

Weintrobe, S. (2021). *Psychological Roots of the Climate Crisis*. London: Bloomsbury Press.

Interruption 7

Jacob

Jacob is lying on a mattress in the school gym. I am standing at a distance, and our eyes meet momentarily. Jacob jumps up, watching me watching him. He steps off the mattress and begins to turn, smooth and controlled, arms outstretched, eyes tracing a circle on the polished, wooden floor, round and round until he stops, facing me. He meets my gaze, and as if reassured that I am attending, he runs with free abandon across the length of the hall, picking up speed as he goes, only stopping at the boundary of the wall where he places the palms of his hands firmly against the magnolia paintwork. He studies the backs of his hands briefly, before flicking his right hand in towards his chest and turning his head to look at me. I remain attentively where I am standing. He runs back across the length of the hall – this time slowly, more like a trot, with his head turned towards me and a smile on his face. He returns to the blue plastic mattress and lies on his stomach, knees bent and feet waving nonchalantly towards the ceiling. Jacob cups his chin in his hands and takes the weight of his head in his elbows that press into the mattress. He looks at me intensely.

Waiting.

I hesitate and then open my arms and turn around once, slowly. I then walk to the back of the room, tracing his pathway, and place my hands on the wall before turning back to look at him. I walk towards the mattress, closing the distance between us and all the time returning Jacob's gaze. As I get near the mattress, I pause, waiting for the next cue. Jacob has been watching me carefully. He begins to bounce his feet on the mattress, with his chin still cupped in his hands, making small indentations with each bounce; I move closer with the intention of sitting next to him.

'Shall I join you on the mattress?' I say.

But before I have time to sit down, Jacob responds by jumping up, standing close and staring intensely at me.

'Oh! It looks like you have come to join me,' I say.

DOI: 10.4324/9781003322658-15

I hold his gaze, noticing the rich brown velvet of his eyes. His body tenses, as if surprised by a gust of freezing wind. His shoulders lift and he stands, pigeon toed, pressing the backs of his hands together and downwards, towards his bent knees. I stand facing him, consciously slowing my rational thinking brain that is seeking the right response as I trust that I can intuit this conversation. In a moment of synchrony, we begin to run slowly, side by side, the length of the room, stopping at the wall and placing the palms of our hands against the weary paintwork. Jacob looks at his hands and then at mine. I notice his brown skin and the callouses on the back of his hand. My skin looks dark pink against the magnolia wall.

'I'm noticing that your hands are different from mine," I say.

He takes his hands off the wall and vocalises a soft, fluted sigh. I follow his initiative, and we begin to play, sometimes synchronising our movement, sometimes contrasting, coming together and acknowledging each other and then moving part. Our feet trace winding pathways on the wooden floor. I sense small changes in Jacob's rhythmic energy, careful to note how his run turns into a gallop and then into a walk.

Jacob comes towards me and tests the ground with an emphatic jump. I stand still. He looks at me and then turns away, his body seeming suddenly frozen, with knees bent and hands clasped. He lifts his nose in the air, reminding me of a young deer smelling danger in the wind. I feel a surge of sadness, as if I am losing him. Facing away from me, Jacob sinks down onto his knees. He crouches down, looking at the floor, and bangs the knuckles of his right hand against the palm of his left hand. Instinctively, I begin to move slowly backwards. As I do so, the intensity of his hand movement lessens.

'Perhaps you need to be alone now,' I say.

It is near the end of the session. I am deeply moved by this brief connection. In my mind's eye, I play with words to reflect the experience, but everything seems inadequate. I vocalise a soft, fluted sigh and noticed an almost imperceptible movement of Jacob's head.

'We need to finish and go back to the classroom,' I say.

I walk over to where we have left our shoes at the beginning of the session. As is usual at the end of Jacob's session, I put my shoes on, stand up and pick up Jacob's shoes. He runs to me, takes his shoes and puts them on. Without looking at each other, or speaking, we head off back to the classroom side by side.

8   Endings

We sit in silence. I am conscious that Maeve sees me glance at the clock. There are 3 minutes more. She reaches into her bag by the side of her chair and brings something out that she stretches towards me.

'I made you this.'

A green velvet purse melts into the palm of my hand. I run my index finger along the detailed embroidery around the edge. The mother-of-pearl button fastening catches the light. Hot tears prick behind my eyes.

'This is beautiful,' I say spontaneously. 'Thank you. I'm really touched.'

I look at Maeve and notice tears pooling in her eyes. Lowering her head, a tear drops into her lap. She straightens her white shirt by pulling its edge down on either side of her torso and shifts back into her seat. I notice newly grown soft curls hugging her skull, and for a moment, she looks like a young boy.

'I was hoping you'd like it,' she says.
    'Hmm,' I nod.

The silent voice in my head says *I do, I really do.* Maeve looks up, and we smile as another tear spills down her cheek. She sniffs and wipes her eyes with the back of her right hand.

'I made it and then I got cold feet. I wasn't sure about bringing it, but then I decided to anyway.'
    'It's a beautiful gift, thank you.'

DOI: 10.4324/9781003322658-16

I imagine Maeve crafting the purse. I picture my late mother's sewing box, with the tapestry lid that hardly closed, bulging with ribbons, attachments, needles, pins, cotton reels, scissors, buttons and scraps of coloured materials that she would skilfully transform into articles and artefacts. I remember the reassuring hum of the sewing machine.

'It was just scraps in the sewing box,' Maeve says.
'It's a work of art,' I respond.
'As I was making it, I was thinking about what I said earlier about how it was scary to be here at first. How I didn't know what to say or what to do. And now, you know, I just turn up and it's OK to be here with . . . whatever . . . I know we're ending, but part of me doesn't want to.'
'Well,' I say, looking at the clock, 'It *is* time to end now and I really wish you well, Maeve . . . out there in the world.'

Maeve picks up her bag, and we walk together to the door of the studio. I feel a pulling sensation in my chest. Maeve opens the door, and in the reception area, she grasps the back of the chair and slips on her shoes. She throws her bag over her shoulder, saying,

'See you then, and thanks again.'

Before I can respond, she makes a hasty exit, closing the outer door behind her. I walk back into the studio and notice that Maeve has left her car keys on the floor by the chair. I smile as I pick up the keys. I put Maeve's gift on the chair and head to the door, to hear Maeve running back. At the door, I hold up the keys, smiling, raising my eyebrows and tilting my head to one side. Maeve has a look of playful delight on her flushed face.

'There you go,' she says, taking the keys and shaking them in the air. 'One last goodbye . . ..'
'Goodbye, Maeve; go well . . .' I say, still holding the door handle with my left hand.

I lift my right hand to wave, but Maeve has disappeared through the outer door without looking back.
The door closes with a bang.
Returning inside the studio, I sense a wave of something inside me that is hard to name. An unsettled feeling in my torso creeps up to my jaw and into the roof of my mouth. I swallow. Outside the window, a blackbird calls into the summer, and I feel alone in this empty, silent studio. I look at Maeve's gift lying on her seat. The jangle of her keys

echoes in my ears. I remember that playful look on her face as she left. I feel bereft and depleted, here, in this studio without Maeve, knowing that she will not return.

Standing on the wooden floor, I take in a breath and push the air out so that it rushes past my lips as I puff out my cheeks. A tear spills down my face. I stretch my arms out either side, as if trying to fill the space. Feeling some tension in my shoulders, I twist my spine to the right and then the left and roll my shoulders, as if something needs releasing. I reach both hands upwards and catch sight of small brown blemishes on the white paintwork of the V-shaped ceiling. It seems a long way up. My eye runs along the beams that stretch across the room, and I picture Maeve's stories of playing in the barn as a child.

Bringing my arms slowly down in front of me to waist level, I take another deep breath in before sighing on the out-breath. I follow an impulse to sway gently from right to left and right again, allowing my arms to follow the line of the movement, like seaweed drifting in the current.

A fluted call of the blackbird breaks the silence.

I stand still and look around the studio, becoming aware of the soft ticking of the clock that veils the silence. The sun creates a rectangular pathway of light that glimmers on the wooden floor in front of my feet. I step into the warmth of the sunlight and notice how my optimism and my fear for Maeve converge in the waters of loss. The absence of my long-gone mother is present like a distant rumble of thunder that echoes through the image of her sewing box.

Endings as entanglements

Maeve and I had reached the end of our agreed time working together. As I sit here now at the laptop remembering my experience of that last session, it becomes entangled with the diffractive unfolding of the end this book. It is early March. There is frogspawn in the pond, and the spring flowers are bringing their colour to the world. Out of the window, a pair of blue tits dances in the entangled branches of the naked wisteria, and the rasping cries of the rooks catch my attention as they make their nests high up in the taller trees beyond. Ironically, the finalising of this book, and thus these words on endings, became interrupted and delayed by the death of my father just a few months before his 100th birthday. In writing the eulogy for his funeral, I found myself tracking the remarkable path of an individual as it unfolded across a century. Endings, like beginnings, diffract within wider matrices of material-discursive entanglements, always in the process of the corporeality of the world's becoming. And you too, as the reader, are located in this entanglement, as we enter this final chapter together. I find myself wondering what you are making of your place in this ending.

Maeve's final departure, as described in this vignette, illustrates how small, spontaneous, intra-active moments unfold within endings that have been thought about over time in the process of the therapeutic work. These final poignant moments were part of an improvised unfolding. Maeve had missed the session 2 weeks previously because of a funeral. Following that absence, the penultimate session had then been an opportunity to reflect on bringing our work to a close, before we arrived into this final goodbye. When Maeve had left and I was by myself, I noticed the immediate impact of that loss and allowed my body a few moments to move into the experience. The reality is that in a busy working day, this kind of processing can be squeezed out as, for example, resources dwindle, workloads intensify and the demands to provide end-to-end sessions, meet organisational targets and produce tangible outputs increase. Without time to slow down, process and feel the impact of our relationships through the receptivity of the moving body, there is a danger that the only way to manage the demands of a workplace becomes emotional detachment, denial and disavowal, rather than allowing time to move through the feelings.

Endings that move through

Endings can take many forms, including difficult complex endings that manifest in the therapeutic relationship, for example, when a client suddenly stops attending through a less conscious acting out, as a defence against thinking about and feeling the impact of previous abrupt losses. I remember a client who had attended sessions regularly, convincingly insisting that in their engagement with previous therapy, they had already processed the trauma of suddenly losing a close teenage friend in an accident. Suddenly and without warning, they left the therapy, and *I* was left holding the difficult and uncomfortable feelings triggered by a brutal and unexpected departure.

During the COVID-19 pandemic, the world found itself moving through unfamiliar landscapes in which losses and endings of many kinds became strongly thematic. Breathing bodies became sites of contamination and suspicion, and there were many abrupt and distressing endings and disruptions. An emphasis on sanitation and social distancing to reduce unnecessary contact, along with obligations, such as keeping rooms ventilated, highlighted our entangled intra-dependency, troubling neoliberal ideas about humans as autonomous and separate individuals. In therapy practice, these losses and endings within the pandemic manifest not least through illness, social restrictions and the complications of shifting from face-to-face to online working.

In my work as a DMP in education, there have been distressing endings, when children or young people have been permanently excluded from school before the therapeutic process is completed, in which case I have needed to use supervision to process all kinds of difficult feelings evoked in me. I have often had to come to terms with being just one small part in the wider, complex and sometimes dysfunctional assemblages of the lives of these children and young people, including systemic injustices and oppressions. As a practitioner, I have needed to find ways of mourning the loss of clients on different levels, and these losses are held deeply within the emotional currents of the moving body, every ending being unique in some way and touching me differently. In some special schools in which I have worked, the death of children and young people in that community sadly has not been an unusual occurrence due to medical and life-limiting conditions, and I have needed to find ways to attend to my own sense of loss, whilst also supporting others in my role as a DMP. Curtis (2017) illustrates how organisational responses to the death of a child in schools can differ, ranging from one in which the devastating impact of the loss is sensitively acknowledged and embraced in the collective mourning of the whole school, to another in which the sadness and grief are defended against by a 'culture of denial' (83) and the school quickly moves on from the loss. In building cultures of care, it is crucial that we allow spaces to move through the feelings that are evoked by the losses that occur on many levels. That *moving through* involves the emotional materiality of the creative improvisational movement, as otherwise, cultures of detachment and denial in the face of loss can result in a collective desensitisation. DMP practitioner Barjacoba-Souto (2023) shares her experiential process of mourning the death of a child with whom she had worked in a special school. The DMP sessions had come to an end months before his death, and having already said good-bye when the clinical work finished, she found herself in a place of grief on hearing subsequently of his death in the community in which she still worked. Barjacoba-Souto describes how she processed this loss through improvisational movement, through which she was able to access the grief that came alive in her body. She begins her improvisation locating her bodied connection with the world around her, writing

> I find myself alone in my living room, a light and airy space. Standing facing a large window, I stare at the sky. I see some clouds, the sun and big trees. The sunrays entering the room appear to be flooding the space whilst a turmoil of emotions start flooding my body.
>
> (173)

As practitioners, we can yearn for particular kinds of (good enough) endings, yet the reality is that as we encounter endings, we are moving through the entanglement of unfolding processes in which each of us is just one presence within complex material-discursive assemblages. Rather than getting caught up in a grandiose sense of our own exceptional power as a practitioner to guide others to a place of resolution, we need to be prepared to immerse ourselves in the specificities of the emotional currents within the waters of intra-active relationships. And at the same time, there is an ethical duty to think carefully about how endings and losses are contained.

The experience of endings and losses can come in many forms. I remember an adult client who was a successful professional, presenting as likeable and confident, with a great sense of humour. Yet they also described how at times they would become struck by a terrible existential anxiety. In one session, they were drawn to the movement space and began to pace urgently across the wooden floor, changing direction seemingly at random, arms pushing through invisible obstacles. Gradually their movement became still, they dropped to their knees, and placing the palms of their hands on the floor, they curled their body into a ball and began to sob. They later described a sense of grief for all the pain and suffering in the world, for environmental degradation and for all the species lost and never to return. In that moment, as they sobbed, all I could do was connect with their despair in solidarity (Frizell, 2023b). It was hard to find words for the emotional intensity of the solidarity between us, and at times, the spontaneous, improvised expression of moving bodies has an intelligence of its own. The intensity of the emotional connection and the experience of solidarity in response to biodiversity loss stayed with me, and some days later, while walking on a country path, I came across a dead badger. I was moved to write the following poem:

Elegy for a Badger

Yesterday,
A badger's body caught my eye at the side of the road, lying in a
pool of blood.

Her nose
stretched towards a clump of wilting snowdrops at the foot of
the hedgerow.
Smooth hair
on her rounded rump was coated in red soil, from fields
sloping gently upwards.

Rolling hills
were peppered with bleating lambs staggering
precariously to their feet.

Somehow, poetry, rather than prose, enabled me to express my sense of injustice at the loss of this beautiful badger who had been hit by a car, contrasted by the newborn lambs staggering to their feet in the adjacent field. Despair and hope sat side by side. It is not always possible to represent and make sense of experiences through rational language, yet the privileging of language over other ways of knowing the world is compelling. Poynor (2023) describes how she processed the death of a friend that was entangled with the difficult experience of attending the funeral via zoom, due to it being conducted on the other side of the world. She describes how she was able to give form to her difficult experience and feelings through improvisational movement and voice whilst witnessed and supported in a peer exchange. The improvised movement itself enabled her to reconnect with her body and her feelings as she traversed her internal chaos, and the experience provided both a catalyst and a container. In her writing, Poynor (ibid) emphasises the importance of

> (f)oregrounding movement itself, not only as a means of exploration and expression, but as a therapeutic medium, a process of re-solving and integrating challenging emotions, personal issues and dilemmas, and psychological tensions. Valuing kinaesthetic intuition and embodied language as alternative ways of knowing and understanding our life experiences. Learning to trust enough to follow what arises in an untrammelled way.
>
> (104)

Poynor argues that we need not, and indeed sometimes cannot, aways reduce creative improvisation to representational language. The value can remain in the poetry of the experience.

When Maeve left the room for the last time, I spent a few moments noticing my own immediate experience of that separation. I found myself experiencing the space as big and empty. Maeve's gift, lying on her seat, was a material reminder of her absence. Sensory memories of the immediate encounter remained with me, such as the jangle of her car keys and the childlike delight that I sensed in her face as she ran back to collect them. The unsettled feeling in my torso, which rose through my jaw and into the top of my mouth, was my sense of bereavement in that empty space where Maeve and I had spent many hours together. We had both risked entering a strong attachment, knowing that this relationship would come to an end within this assemblage. As I stepped into the warmth of the sunlight, I noticed how my optimism and my fear for Maeve converged with my sense of loss as this relationship ended. Maeve's gift had evoked memories of my own mother, and maternal loss was a prevalent theme in this encounter. This was a complex entanglement.

Endings as poetry

In my ending with Maeve, two (post)human moving bodies were immersed in material-discursive entanglements that shapeshifted in *spacetimemattering* unfoldings, that is, as space, time and matter intra-acted and diffracted through the poetry of this ending. The creative force that brings relational bodies into places of becoming hovers in every mo(ve)ment, and the improvisation arising from that creativity offers a relational language of experience. These are the lungs that breathe life into the poetry of existence. In the same way that words conjure stories, that sound transforms into music and that art manifests in structural forms, so the materiality of a world in movement can transform into dance.

As Maeve and I closed our work together, there were many actors:

the clock   two women   a handmade purse   women's voices
     a mother of pearl button   hot tears   studio space
Maeve's newly grown hair   a white shirt   a glance   affection
     wooden floor   uncertainty   sunlight and shadows
the hum of a sewing machine   doors opening and closing   playful delight
     jangling keys   sadness   the fluted call of the blackbird
a v-shaped ceiling   joy   swaying   my mother's sewing box   humour
     stretching   twisting   drifting   reaching   blemished paintwork
the rush of the outbreath   a wooden beam   silence (but for) a ticking clock

The relational connections between each element created the poetry of this lived experience of ending. Feminist philosopher and physicist Barad (2007) reminds us that moving (human) bodies are just one part of the world's differential performative affect economy, rather than being independently situated within a passive material world. Material bodies of all kin(ds) affected and were affected within this rhizomatic assemblage, and as each element bumped up against another, possibilities for new narratives were becoming created. Maeve had discovered a confidence in navigating the unknown, the uncertain and the unplanned and, as such, had become more able to *just turn up* into this rhizomatic assemblage without a preconceived idea of what would unfold. The potential of this intra-active dynamic space between material-discursive things is the diffractive playing space (Winnicott, 1971) that is contingent and indeterminant. Within new materialist and posthuman thought, this relational space moves away from a human-centric focus to include a more diverse range of agentic actors that move through rhizomatic flows of intensities.

Endings as flows of intensities

As I now describe the 3 minutes of my final session with Maeve, I am illustrating '*practices of attuning* to embodied intensities' (Fullagar, 2021: 120) that emerged within the relational entanglements of this assemblage and constellated in this ending. My attunement to these embodied intensities depended upon that which I privileged as I listened. That is, the choices that I made (consciously and less consciously) about what I chose to give attention to, that what I filtered out, what I held onto as significant, what I chose to share explicitly and what I chose to leave unsaid. As a practitioner, I moved continuously through flows of intensities, making decisions about how it might be useful to respond to Maeve, whilst allowing a playful spontaneity to unfold. For example, when Maeve states that she was hoping that I liked the gift, there was a desperate voice inside me that wanted to reassure her that *I do, I really do* that I resisted. Then the vivid image of my late mother's sewing box indicated that Maeve had touched a deeply personal place in me that connected to the creativity of maternal holding. I did not consider that it would have been helpful to share these thoughts and images with Maeve; however, the richness of their symbolism was powerful, and this gave shape to the flows of emotional intensity that became created within the intra-action, mediated through the exchange of a gift.

Endings as gifting

When I was studying to be a DMP practitioner, I remember the issues of gifts being mooted in a supervision group. I remember listening attentively to strongly opinionated oppositional perspectives about whether or not a practitioner should accept a gift from a client. If the therapist does not accept the gift, how can this be done with compassion and in service to the process of the client. If the practitioner does accept a gift, how can this be thought about symbolically within the client's process. If a practitioner has an urge to give a client a gift of some kind, how can this be thought about, and is it always an acting out? Over the years, I have come to realise that what is most important is that any such action is thought about with utmost care, rather than developing a formula for right and wrong. Either way, the exchange of gifts, or even the idea of exchanging gifts, constitutes a symbolic enactment. Maeve offered me her gift 3 minutes before the end of the last session, which did not allow any time to process the exchange. I chose to accept Maeve's gift, and in those 3 remaining minutes of our time together, the gift served as a catalyst for an emotional exchange in which Maeve's experience, her expression and her presence diffracted with my own (her) stories. In fostering my capacity to listen sensitively and responsively, I took responsibility for my participatory role in this assemblage, remaining alert to the dancer in me and engaging my '(m)yriad tentacles' (Haraway, 2016: 31) of emotional, sensory, intellectual and intuitive perceptions that moved through lines of flight, moments of diffraction and flows of intensity.

Ending actively

Maeve's insightful observation that she had been increasingly able *just to turn up* was part of a wider narrative of the performativity of identity politics, as well as the micro-moments of relational connectivity that unfolded between us over time. During the process of the therapy, Maeve had explored her experience as a working-class, migrant woman and mother entering menopause. Her confidence in her entitlement to turn up and claim the space had been crushed in systemic oppressions. As the therapist, I needed to watch out for and monitor my own place of privilege, as well as my own experience of oppression and injustice that infused the flows of intensity within the less conscious dynamics of the transference and the countertransference into which Maeve and I both turned up, and that turned up between us. Thank goodness for supervision! As we finished, I sensed that Maeve was now better able to withstand this intra-personal space created between us, and she had realised a greater confidence in her capacity to participate (just turn up) in this affective matrix, along with a better understanding of the performativity of oppressions and injustices. In this way, therapy itself becomes a form of activism that enables clients to unpack their experience within a clearer critique of the socio-political inscriptions that have become internalised and performed on micro, mezzo and macro levels. The lens of intersectionality can be helpful in realising the power differentials that move through social identities that make it harder for some people to turn up than others, depending on their sense of entitlement and assumptions about privilege and belonging that have become internalised.

At the time of this ending, there was a lot going on in Maeve's life. She was moving house and starting a new job. She had also begun spending more time with the craft-making that she loved. Maeve seemed better equipped to know that she could manage the vicissitudes of life, and she had rediscovered the power of creativity and play. She was also better able to identify and refuse enactments of her internalised subordination. Maeve seemed to have developed the confidence to step into the rhizomatic entanglements of attachments and losses that would bring her to the edge of new possibilities and potential. Those edges can seem like difficult places. As a therapist, I am alert to potential enactments (theirs and mine) in the less conscious narratives that get played out. For example, if clients bring stories of difficult endings, such as the sudden or traumatic death of someone close, or an experience of being abandoned, I listen to those stories wondering about the possibility of enactments in the immediate relationship. I invite a processing of some of the more difficult feelings that are potentially kept at bay by an acting out within the emerging attachment.

Endings through attachments and losses

Attachments and losses are intra-subjective, relational processes of connectivity in which bodies of all kin(ds) are emergent and entangled within multi-dimensional assemblages. Processes of forming attachments and withstanding separations and losses, of holding on and letting go, and of arriving and departing comprise diffractive encounters within potential spaces of *becoming* that are live and dynamic. Conceptually and experientially, beginnings and endings imply that meaningful attachments and losses are happening in relation to, for example, another person, another creature, a material thing, a stage in life, a way of life, states of health and well-being, places or landscapes, beliefs, ideas or experiences and more. Mabey (2005) describes his debilitating depression that followed the completion of an all-consuming nature writing project. Once the project was over and the book published, he experienced a tremendous sense of loss and emptiness. His writing tracks his slow recovery from a terrible depression as he rekindled his love and relational connection within both the human world and the earth.

I have worked with many students who attend higher education institutions in the UK from overseas who have left their families, friends and their homelands. Along with missing families and friends, the loss of, for example, landscapes and animals is also felt acutely. I have been deeply moved by stories of the painful longing of an overseas student to be reconnected with the family dog. Levine (2005) describes loss as 'the absence of something we were once attached to,' (9) and I wonder about the different kinds of attachments and losses that you can identify from your own experience, and what those attachments tell you about what it is that you privilege and prioritise and where it is that you find kinship.

Jungian analyst Jerome Bernstein (2005) identified what he describes as *borderland* clients, who experience strong feelings of despair in the face the loss of connection with the earth that is inherent in our Western post-industrial, advanced capitalist culture. He describes a client who talks of carrying a 'Great Grief' (ibid 73), which is an intimate part of himself as he mourns the losses of environmental degradation felt on a deeply personal level. When we have a deep kinship (aka attachment) with the earth's ecology, environmental degradation is then felt as a personal loss.

The things with which we create attachments are those things with which we find kinship, that is, the matter(s) that has(ve) come to matter.

Endings in kinship

It is now impossible to ignore climate chaos as a context for our lives, and the loss of biodiversity is very real. The climate is changing. Species are disappearing. Homelands are threatened. The future is uncertain. We live the loss. Increasingly, therapists are integrating ideas about environmental awareness, in terms of the existential threat that can present as eco-anxiety and, also, in terms of conceptualising human subjectivity as an intra-dependent phenomenon within a wider ecology. Earth is our home, and the strong attachments to that earth as home manifest in our sense of empathic resonance and kinship within that ecology. Creative moving bodies have the potential to call worlds into relationship. This relational dancing then has the potential to enter the stage of transversal subjectivities in which kinship is found in the dynamic and empathic meeting places of differences.

It is important that an attitude of care underpins our relationships in each moment. However, within our current economic system, those in the caring professions can find low paid, casualised contracts are the norm; caring being associated with a low economic value. An increasingly pervasive neoliberal ideology commodifies people and well-being within the care industry. The lived experiences of care providers and those receiving care can be one of fragmentation, unrest and inequality. These inequalities within the care sector became magnified as the COVID-19 pandemic unfolded. Structural discriminations surfaced, as, for example, we discovered that learning-disabled adults were 30 times more likely to die from COVID-19 than the general population, and, in addition, *Do Not Resuscitate* orders were justified simply by someone having a learning disability (Tapper, 2021).

The neoliberal hegemony of the relentless progression of advanced capitalism has resulted in inequalities that are devastating for many. A boon time for the super-rich sits alongside brutal austerity measures in health, social, community and voluntary service provision. Professionals struggle with dwindling resources, which can lead to burnout and emotional disconnection. It becomes increasingly difficult to practise with care and integrity in the face of managerialism, as well as in the face of demands for number-crunching, positivist outcome measures (Frizell, 2023c). Like other arts psychotherapies, DMP practice as a mental health provision might be measured against performance targets, and in such an atmosphere, provision can become dehumanised and soulless, resulting in practitioners operating in a state of disavowal (Skaife & Martyn, 2022). Hayes (2013) wonders how care contexts can become places of enchantment, in which there is a duty of care to keep the soul and spirit alive and a duty of policymakers, managers and practitioners to foster empathy and kinship. We have a duty to care about caring, and we need to refuse systemic failures of care whereby efficient use of resources take precedence over the lives of individuals in frameworks of un-care (Weintrobe, 2021). Coming home into our ecofeminist, posthuman, new materialist bodies brings us (as practitioners and clients) into complex entangle-ments of material-discursive phenomena that are infused with 'a hopefulness that enables us to care and a carefulness that enables us to hope' (Frizell, 2023a: 77). Cultures of care become entangled with our experiences of endings and loss.

Ending care-fully

As practitioners and researchers, our work needs to be brought into a twenty-first-century context of the complexities of advanced capitalism that includes social, political, economic and environmental inequalities and injustices. I sug-gest that, as practitioners, we have a duty to remain abreast of those inequalities and injustices in an ongoing critique of the systemic creation and perpetuation of binaries of dominion and subordination. Now, more than ever, there is an ethical imperative to shift from binaries into multiplicities towards transversal subjectivities (Braidotti, 2019). These perspectives have been operational for me in resisting and critiquing the hierarchical ranking of bodies through medi-cal, political, social, educational, cultural and environmental discourses, return-ing again and again to the different possibilities of moving-bodies-politic(s). As an ecofeminist, researching-practitioner and practising-researcher, this critique continuously simmers in my orbit of awareness, ready to bubble up into acts of resistance. In this writing, I am illustrating how ethico-onto-epistemologies of new materialism and posthumanism have enabled me to move through com-plexities of material-discursive phenomena. In short, I strive as an ecofeminist, researching-practitioner and practising-researcher to move with the deepest re-lational respect for the *other* as moving bodies enter the performative connectiv-ity of material-discursive worlds. As flowers blossom in vibrant blue or yellow; as horses run, jump and roll in fields or as silver slow-worms slither under grass cuttings, so dance practising offers humans a relational, empathic contingent potential space ripe for practising alternative corporealities, in which attach-ments, losses and kinship can find new ways to move through our complex intra-dependence.

The musings in the chapters of this book seek to optimise the potential of how kinship might be imagined and performed through relational moving bodies within climates of equality and justice. The values and principles that we bring to our work as ecofeminist researching-practitioners and practising-researchers can illuminate and animate (intra-)subjectivities differently towards creating environments that are welcoming, rather than hostile.

It has not been my intention in this book to create a new paradigm for practice and research but rather to illustrate how, identifying as an ecofeminist, I have brought the lenses of new materialism, posthumanism and their inherent principles of intersectionality to my work. The book is a contribution to a body of work that supports an orientation to ways in which practitioners, researchers and educators can think differently about how identities are organised and subjectivities performed. I value psychodynamic principles, along with their potential to hold the contradictions and complexities of inner world, relational experiences. Critical lenses can enhance and challenge these principles, shedding new light on both the theory and the practice, for example, of object relations, transference and countertransference, attachment and loss, projection and defences.

Ending diffractively and inconclusively

I close this book (for now), stepping into gratitude as an act of resistance that refuses the exceptionalism that creates hierarchies of worth and refuses elitist entitlements. This gratitude takes nothing for granted and shapeshifts within the diffractive moving waves created by all things. Gratitude as a form of activism creates a space to pause, think and decouple from human exceptionalism and entitlement that drives a neoliberal agenda. My hope is that this book reaches out into the wider landscapes of the caring professions. I suggest that the ideas that unfold through material-discursive dancing bodies can serve as multiple springboards to inspire you to foster your own research and practice, keeping in touch with your curious and creative moving bodies, whilst simultaneously moving through critical discourses. In this way, love, care, compassion and empathy can be threaded through each diffractive moment of intra-action. Ecofeminist DMP and ecopsychotherapy, with posthumanism and new materialism at their heart, can inspire researcher-practitioners and practitioner-researchers to move within relational networks of material-discursive properties that make for multiple relational possibilities.

To finish, I step into a movement space.

I am pacing. I am p(l)acing (with) a foot, placing an arm and (p)lacing the mo(ve)ment before sinking to the floor. I discover myself buried under the sand. Sand above me, below me and beside me. As I shift my position, different parts of me appear above the sand.

And disappear.

A sand hopper springs off the ground in a sudden burst of energy.

And another.

I shift my movement with and as sand. Lifting and revealing parts of my body and shifting back into my sand-creature self. Finding my orientation in the world through tiny (grains of) sand (creatures). Disappearing and then coming into (my) existence.

My movement is fluid and sequential and increasingly slow, although it doesn't stop. There is life running through the currents of my slowing movement, and the texture of the air changes.

It thickens.

It thins.

It becomes infused with other ways of being. And the floor speaks to me, pushing me from one place to the other. I contact the floor, and it contacts me back and directs my movement.

Slowly I begin to rise.

Evolving upwards, first on four legs, lifting my body slightly off the ground. Then curving and crawling before lifting my weight onto two legs. And then the straightening of the spine brings me into a human (well, a certain kind of human) who experiences verticality on two feet.

A word comes . . .

. . . so . . .

. . . and others . . . . . . even . . .

. . . though . . .

. . . is it?. . .

. . . can it? . . .

. . . I (don't) know . . . . . . hold this (a) moment . . .

Between the words, the movement flows through me, from one side to another and into a spiral. I am reaching (out) into (from) the outside–inside world. I pull the outside world (towards me). I try to hold on (to it), balancing on one leg, arms curving around. Moving slowly, unaware of the breath that is always going on.

More words erupt . . .

. . . even though . . .

. . . but . . .

. . . perhaps . . .

The words burst (out) into the space of their own volition, as conjunctions that hold an interest between one thought and another. Words that fill the wordlessness in the dance and float suspended in the air. I move to one edge of the room to look in from the outside, with my back against the wall (is that the inside?) as if pretending to objectify the world as a thing. But this wall tells me that there is something excluded from this space on the other side of the wall behind me.

With my back against the wall, I look into this (in)conclusion. Into this end. Into this disappearance.[1] And in that disappearance is my subjectivity.

I lean back into the wall.

Rising on my toes, I balance, now steadied by the back of my head pushing against the wall as my spine is released. I am suspended until my elbow replaces that point of contact. Then the tip of my finger on the wall steadies my balance before I step forwards, into this (in)conclusion, that is the end.

'It's time.'

I am and it is (never) finished.

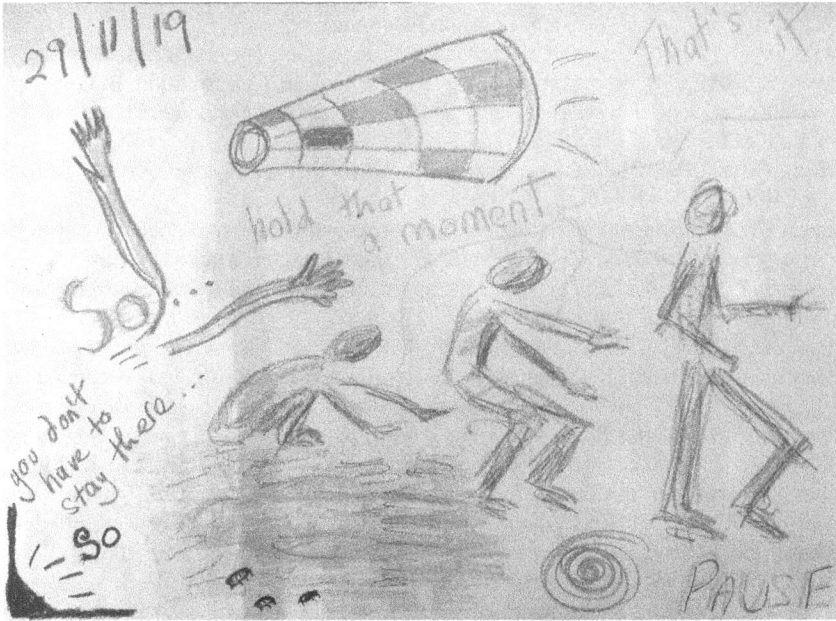

Figure 8.1 Human of sorts.

Provocation

What are the endings and losses that are with you as you finish this book?
    I invite you to honour one of those endings through improvised dance, art, music, theatre, poetry or some other form of creative expression.
    Find a trusted colleague, friend, peer, etc., with whom to share that creation.

Note

1 This improvisation manifest as I was beginning the research process on which this book was based in autumn 2019. With hindsight, I realise that in looking into the beginning, I was looking towards this (in)conclusion. The illustration, Figure 28, A Human of Sorts, pp. 138, was a response to the movement improvisation.

References

Barad, K. (2007). *Meeting the Universe Halfway: Quantum Physics and the Entanglement of Matter and Meaning*. London: Duke University Press.

Barjacoba-Souto, B. (2023). Dancing with Stephen: Reconnecting with the body in a search for closure. In C. Frizell and M. Rova (eds.), *Creative Bodies in Therapy, Performance and Community Research and Practice that Brings Us Home*, pp. 171–179. London: Routledge.

Bernstein, J. (2005). *Living in the Borderland: The Evolution of Consciousness and the Challenge of Healing Trauma*. London: Routledge.

Braidotti, R. (2019). *Posthuman Knowledge*. Cambridge: Polity Press.

Curtis, S. (2017). On becoming a monkey. In G. Unkovich, C. Butte and J. Butler (eds.), *Dance Movement Psychotherapy with People with Learning Disabilities*, pp. 81–93. Oxon: Routledge.

Frizell, C. (2023a). Bodies, landscapes, and the air that we breathe. *Kritika Kultur*, Vol. 40, pp. 66–73.

Frizell, C. (2023b). Coming home to a posthuman body; Finding hopefulness in those who care. In D. Parker, C. Jackson and L. Aspey (eds.), *Holding the Hope: Reviving/restoring Psychological and Spiritual Agency in the Face of Climate Change*, pp. 76–85. Monmouth: PCCS Books.

Frizell, C. (2023c). The cat, the foal and other meetings that make a difference: Posthuman research that re-animates our responsiveness to knowing and becoming. In C. Frizell and M. Rova (eds.), *Creative Bodies in Therapy, Performance and Community Research and Practice that Brings Us Home*, pp. 50–61. London: Routledge.

Fullager, S. (2021). Re-turning to embodied matters and movement. In K. Murris (ed.), *Navigating the Post Qualitative New Materialist and Critical Posthumanist Terrain Across Disciplines: An Introductory Guide*, pp. 117–134. Oxon: Routledge.

Haraway, D. (2016). *Staying with the Trouble*. London: Duke University Press.

Hayes, J. (2013). *Soul and Spirit in Dance Movement Psychotherapy: A Transpersonal Approach*. London: Jessica Kingsley.

Levine, (2005). *Unattended Sorrow: Recovering from Loss and Reviving the Heart*. USA: Holtzbrinck Publishers.

Mabey, R. (2005). *Nature Cure*. London: Random House.

Poynor, H. (2023). Is that yoga or are you just making it up?. In C. Frizell and M. Rova (eds.), *Creative Bodies in Therapy, Performance and Community Research and Practice that Brings Us Home*, pp. 101–108. London: Routledge.

Skaife, S. and Martyn, J. (2022). *Art Psychotherapy Groups in the Hostile Environment of Neoliberalism*. London: Routledge.

Tapper, J. (2021). Fury at 'do not resuscitate' notices given to Covid patients with learning disabilities. *The Guardian*, Saturday 13th February, 13.56GMT. www.theguardian.com/world/2021/feb/13/new-do-not-resuscitate-orders-imposed-on-covid-19-patients-with-learning-difficulties

Weintrobe, S. (2021). *Psychological Roots of the Climate Crisis*. London: Bloomsbury Press.

Winnicott, D. W. (1971). *Playing and Reality*. London: Tavistock.

Epilogue

Existential wonderings and wanderings

Samhain is approaching as they set out, rucksacks filled with cheese and onion sandwiches, wet weather gear and bottles of water. They stride purposefully past the golden sands of St Ives, as surfers in wet suites gather to catch the incoming tide under grey clouds.

They take the winding coastal path towards Zennor – uneven, rocky and muddy from recent rain. She avoids domes of fresh cowpats lying on the path and cautiously distributes her weight as she moves from one foot to the other, being careful not to slip, noting the skid marks as a reminder. She acknowledges the ghosts of long-gone walkers who gaze out from boot tread patterns in the mud.

To her left, the rocky ground slopes steeply upwards. Purple-flowering heather is dotted amongst bold yellow gorse. The brown ferns are dying back after the summer. A murmuration of linnets catch her attention, and she stops to watch their undulating collective wave. To her right, geometric rocks drop sharply down to the shore, where grey-black boulders lie higgledy-piggledy before the rolling sea. A lone seal swims in a cove below, and the haunting whistles of oyster catchers ride on the wind.

Conscious of being less nimble than before, she senses her vulnerability in this unforgiving landscape. Her mind turns to her nonagenarian father, and she muses on how frailty creeps up unannounced with age, in a way that is unimaginable to the young and strong. Fine rain falls, and she lifts the hood of her raincoat over her head. As she clambers over irregular boulders that line the steep, downwards-winding pathway, she becomes aware of how she can no longer take strength and balance for granted. She feels a sense of loss and shame underneath her wavering confidence in her younger self's assurance that were she to be thrown off-balance, she could catch her fall and continue unharmed. On turning the corner towards yet another steep slope down to the coastline and up again, a wall of wind pushes her back. She opens her arms and releases the weight of her body forwards into the strength of the wind, laughing out loud in a moment of liberation. Still smiling, she strides out, pushing against the force of the wind. Her hood is blown back off her head.

The rain clouds race across the sky, opening curtains on patches of blue. To her right, a cautionary sign states: *Beware: Mine Shafts. Keep to Coastal Path.*

They settle on a granite rock for lunch. He points out a large irregular rock balanced precariously on two smaller rocks on the promontory opposite. She turns to face the wind to eat her sandwich so that her hair blows away from her face. A young couple passes by with heavy rucksacks covered in luminous orange and yellow rain covers. They look up at the two older walkers who are carefully unwrapping the silver foil around their cheese and onion sandwiches in the ferocious wind.

'Found a sheltered spot then,' the man shouts up to them.

They all laugh with a shared sense of adventure.

After the brief stop for lunch, they muster their agility to navigate further rocks, boulders and undulating inclines. On an upwards slope, they come across that same young couple who are now huddled beneath a rock, eating *their* lunch. They all share a smile.

She wills her knees to hold out as they tackle another steep slope downwards leading to a wooden bridge and then they clamber upwards through some boulders, across another wooden bridge and then up some steps carved into the hillside to arrive in open scrubland.

A sign to Zennor welcomes them off the coastal path towards the warm open fire of the Tinners Arms to wait for the taxi back to St Ives.

'You made it then,' says a man on an adjacent table, whose children sit nearby with coke, sweets and crisps.

She remembers passing them on the pathway.

'You kids have done well,' she says, smiling at the ruddy-faced children, who beam back, munching sugar-coated chocolate eggs that have been poured into a pint glass.

This was a family pilgrimage, the man explains, for a father-in-law who, despite a serious illness, has insisted on walking this coastal path, perhaps for the last time.

'He should be here in a bit,' he says, glancing expectantly back at the door.

A member of staff carries in some logs to feed the fire.

Their taxi arrives. As they get in, she sees a group of women, linking arms on either side of a frail, elderly man. They are coming off the coastal path towards the Tinners Arms. She now remembers having passed them on the pathway. As the taxi drives off, she watches this fellow traveller complete what

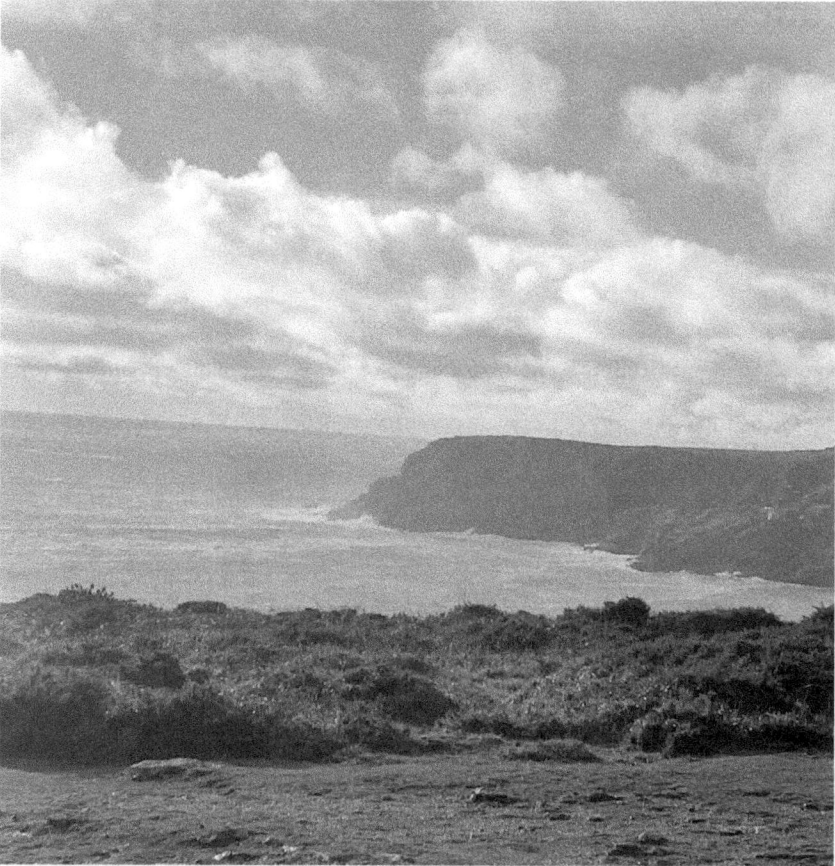

Figure 9.1 St Ives to Zennor.

Source: Photograph by the author.

might have been his final trip on the coastal path from St Ives to Zennor that he loves so dearly.

'St Ives, please!'

The taxi pulls away and turns the corner into the wilderness. The Tinners Arms is out of sight.

Index

Note: Page numbers in *italics* indicate a figure on the corresponding page.

terminology, creating 33–34
racticingization 109; term 35n6
Thatcher's economic revolution 121
therapeutic relationship 6, 82, 103, 130, 144
thing-power 8
time 19n2, 35n7, 46, 125, 147
Toole, David 47, 53n5
transference 103; less conscious
      dynamics 149; racticing through
      less conscious 127–128
transversal subjectivity 34
trust 103

University of London 13, 19n2, 103

Vitruvian Man (da Vinci) 61, 69n2
Voice of the Earth, The (Roszak) 81

Weintrobe, Sally 85
welfare reform 51
well-being 7, 18, 67, 81, 91–92, 132,
    150, 151
Winnicott, Donald 65
Woodger, David 107, 116n4
Work that Reconnects, The
    (programme) 85
Worlding 133; concept of 86;
    as immersion in the world
    32, 137n2; as practice
    principle 133; process
    of 114

Zennor 1, 2, 110, 157–158, *159*

For Product Safety Concerns and Information please contact our EU
representative GPSR@taylorandfrancis.com
Taylor & Francis Verlag GmbH, Kaufingerstraße 24, 80331 München, Germany

41598CB00088B/4254

www.ingramcontent.com/pod-product-compliance
Lightning Source LLC
Chambersburg PA
CBHW060449240326

* 9 7 8 1 0 3 2 3 4 5 3 7 6 *